# HANDS OFF
# MY FOOD!

How Government and Industry Have Corrupted Our Food
and Easy Ways to Fight Back

By

Dr. Sina McCullough

Edited by Lynellen Perry and Janet Smith
Cover Design © Bonnie Watson. All rights reserved.
Author Photo by Julie Massie © www.juliemassie.com All rights reserved.

*Dedicated to my children~*

When darkness surrounds you on all sides,
look inside yourself and you will find your way back home.

**Special Thank You To:**

*My husband–*
For putting up with my crazy ideas,
like when I said I wanted to write a book!
Thank you for never trying to change me.

*Janet Smith–*
For helping me find my voice.

*Dr. Larry Schweikart–*
For helping me learn to trust myself.

*Dr. Peter Osborne–*
For giving me the gift of time.

*Steven Druker, Robert Cohen, Peter Hardin–*
For reviewing my work and providing emotional support.

*Nina Teicholz, Peter Hardin, Jeffrey Smith, Dr. Samuel Epstein, Dr. Tom O'Bryan, Steven Druker, Robert Cohen, Mike Adams–*
For paving the way.

**Through God, this book was possible.**

**Warning:**

This is not a diet book.

The information contained within this book is not meant
to be medical advice nor is it designed to replace advice, information,
or prescriptions you receive from your health care provider.

This book is about an idea.

While I provide solutions, they are suggestions and not advice.

Proceed at your own risk.

# CONTENTS

**Section 3:**
*Easy Ways To Fight Back*

# INTRODUCTION

How much do you know about your food?

Did you know that artificial dye is sometimes added to oranges to make them appear orange?[1] Or that Mountain Dew® contains a flame retardant?[2] And, that ground-up insects are used to make some ketchup look red?[3] Have you heard that some fast food hamburgers contain meat "filler" that is washed in ammonia?[4,5]

What if I told you that companies create synthetic chemicals in laboratories that are put in our processed foods without safety testing and without the FDA's approval or oversight? It's true.[6] Some packaged cake mixes and frostings contain the same ingredient that is used in antifreeze,[7] while some cereals contain a chemical used in jet fuel and embalming fluid.[8-10] Even organic foods can contain dangerous chemicals, which we will discuss in section two of this book. The FDA knows all of this, and they say it's not their problem.[11]

If these facts surprise you, you're not alone. I didn't know any of this until I was forced to learn the truth about our food supply to save my own life. I have a Ph.D. in Nutrition from the University of California at Davis, so I'm technically an "expert" in food. Yet, I ended up getting sick, really sick, from our food. Doctors couldn't figure out what was wrong with me. I saw one specialist after another who performed one test after the next. Nobody had any answers. So, I became my own investigative journalist.

I spent over four years intently studying what's really in our food and how it got there. Sadly, this is the reality we face:

America has a food problem.

**Our food supply is tainted.**

It's making us sick.

We're not only sicker with food-related illnesses like heart disease and autoimmune diseases, **we're losing our freedom**. For example, Americans unknowingly drank experimental milk for nearly eight years in the 1980's.[12] That milk made us sick, and the government knew about it.[13] In fact, our government not only knew, they sanctioned it! To this day, the government continues to offer us up as un-consenting guinea pigs to chemical companies. We'll discuss all of that, in addition to how the government nudges us to choose foods that are making us sick. But, let's first ask ourselves a fundamental question:

Who's responsible for us getting sicker and for the erosion of our freedom?

Some people blame the food industry and call for more government intervention to fix the food problem. Yes, industry played a major role in helping to create the current mess that is our food supply, but they are not the root of the problem. Others blame the government for creating this mess. Yes, government played a role, but it is not the root of the problem either. So, who is the *root* of the problem?

**I am the root of the problem.**
You are the root of the problem.
**"We the People" are the *root* of the problem.**

We've abdicated our responsibility as watchdogs over our food supply. We, the consumers, have allowed ourselves to be lulled into a false sense of security regarding the safety and integrity of our food. Disagree? When was the last time you read an ingredient label, *actually* read the ingredient label, not just glanced at how much fat is listed on the side of the package? When was the last time you questioned if the synthetic chemicals in your favorite box of cookies have been tested for safety?

Many Americans blindly trust our food supply. We eat the food that is sold on the grocery store shelves and don't question it. After all, if the government allows the food to be sold in our stores, it *must* be safe, right? If a company puts chemicals in our food that are used in embalming fluid and jet fuel and the government allows it, they *must* be safe, right? Surely *someone* is making sure these chemicals are safe for us to eat, right?

I used to believe that. I used to blindly trust our food supply. I didn't even realize how much I trusted our food until I was debilitatingly ill.

Since you are reading this book, you are probably already aware that something is wrong with our food supply. You may be looking for solutions. Or, you may be at the beginning of your journey. Regardless of the starting point, this book is designed to help you reach the next step in your journey. This is not a book about blame.

This is a book about finding solutions.

The purpose of this book is to reveal what's really going on with our food supply so we can work together to fix it. As we learn the truth, and each of us takes individual responsibility for our part, that's when the magic happens. That's when the solution becomes clear.

I am the solution.<br>You are the solution.<br>"We the People" are the solution.

Our food supply is a reflection of how we spend our dollars. Consequently, we created our food supply. Once we accept that responsibility, we become empowered. We created it; we can fix it. The good news is that the solution is simple: To restore the integrity of our food supply we must recognize and harness the power we have as consumers.

All we have to do is consciously speak with our dollars.

When it comes to our food supply, I believe we can rally together behind a common goal. That may seem impossible, but it's not. Food should be a unifying issue. Food crosses party lines and political boundaries. After all, we all eat food. We all *need* food. We don't have to agree about what should be in our food supply or on our dinner plates. Just because I don't eat genetically modified organisms (GMOs) or pesticides doesn't mean you can't. Those are individual decisions that each of us can make for ourselves. However, I believe we can find common ground:

- Can we agree that Americans should not be un-consenting guinea pigs for chemical companies?
- Can we agree that government should not decide what's on our dinner plate based on special interest groups and backdoor deals?
- Can we agree that industry should be held accountable when they dump untested synthetic chemicals into our food?
- Can we agree that "We the People" have the right to know what's in the food we eat, even though industry and the FDA are working hard to keep us in the dark?

If we can agree on those points then we have already found common ground. Here is my proposal:

**Let's unite around the idea of individual freedom.**

I would rather decide what's on my dinner plate than have a corporation or the government make that decision for me. I refuse to be an un-consenting guinea pig any longer. I refuse to allow the food industry and the government to keep me in the dark for even one more minute. Let's become an informed citizenry. Then, and only then, can we stand together united by the idea of individual freedom.

My hope is that one day, each of us will go to a grocery store or a fast food chain and know what we are saying with our dollars. I hope that one day, you and I will select our foods based on knowing what's in it, who made it, and whom we are supporting. Making informed decisions is the only way we are going to restore the integrity of our food supply. As you will realize during our time together, industry is not going to fix our food supply, Congress is not going to fix our food supply, and neither are the FDA, USDA, or the EPA. It's up to us, "We the People." We are the ones who will fix the problem. To do that, we need to become an informed citizenry.

**"Educate and inform the whole mass of the people…**
**They are the only sure reliance for the preservation of our**
**liberty."**

—Thomas Jefferson, Letter to Uriah Forrest,
dated December 31, 1787

SECTION 1:


# RECOGNIZING YOUR POWER

# CHAPTER 1:

# DEBILITATINGLY SICK

I blindly trusted our food supply until I became debilitatingly sick. I thought food was safe to eat if I bought it in the grocery store or ordered it off a menu at a restaurant.

After all, we have an entire government agency, the Food and Drug Administration (FDA), which is paid with our tax dollars to look out for our food. I didn't know exactly what they did, but I knew they were watching over my food so that I didn't have to. And, I thought they regulated the food industry so if a company put something bad in my food, the FDA was there to stop them. So, why would I question the safety of our food with our government watchdog on duty?

Besides, the FDA appeared to be doing its job. People weren't routinely getting sick from eating the foods sold in our grocery stores or keeling over in the streets after eating at restaurants. Sure, there was an occasional news report about an *E. Coli* outbreak from spinach contamination resulting in a handful of people getting sick for a few days. But, I viewed those incidents as an excuse to not force myself to eat spinach. Besides, these incidents were "breaking news," which implied the FDA was doing its job.

The FDA and the USDA do a good job of helping to minimize *acute* illnesses that stem from our food supply, like food poisoning. And, to their credit, consumers are aware of the short-term health issues that can arise from food, and they respond accordingly. For example, in 2015 Chipotle® had an *E. Coli* outbreak. Sixty people across eleven states got sick from eating at Chipotle® between October and November. Government health officials and Chipotle's® food safety partner,

IEH Laboratories®, responded almost immediately. They tested surfaces in Chipotle® restaurants to locate the source of the outbreak. Over 3,000 tests were conducted. Consumers responded by not buying food from Chipotle® and sales dropped for the first time in Chipotle® history. Some stores suffered a 15% drop in sales, costing Chipotle® over $72 million in revenue during the 4th quarter. Chipotle® responded to the decrease in consumer confidence by closing stores for half a day to focus on providing their employees with additional training on food safety. In addition, they offered a free burrito to all patrons to get them to return to their stores. It worked; sales increased.[1]

This is an example of how well our current food system works in terms of managing acute or short-term health issues stemming from our food supply. Companies, government, and consumers are knowledgeable and they respond appropriately. The marketplace works in these cases.

### But, how well does our system work when it comes to protecting our *long-term* health?

I'm talking about health issues related to our long-term exposure to our food supply, like what happened to me. My symptoms began in my early 20s. I experienced cramping and bloating within 20 minutes after eating a meal, which was followed by constipation. I knew the problem came from the food I ate. It came from our food supply. But, there didn't seem to be any rhyme or reason behind which foods were causing my pain and which were not. For instance, I could eat a slice of pizza one day and have no problems. The next week I could eat a slice of pizza from the same company and suffer from sharp and painful cramps.

After two months, I sought help from medical doctors. The first doctor I saw recommended I take a prescription drug called Tagamet® with every meal. I was only 20 years old. I was not willing to become dependent on a drug to be able to eat. So, I sought a second opinion, and a third, and a fourth. Eventually, I saw so many primary care doctors and GI specialists that I lost count. I had three colonoscopies, a sigmoidoscopy, two endoscopies, several breath tests for bacterial overgrowth and food sensitivities, too many blood draws, fecal tests, and even exploratory surgery. Twice they found precancerous polyps in my colon, with no known etiology. Nobody knew what was wrong.

Since the doctors could not explain my symptoms, they repeatedly prescribed antibiotics. They assumed I must have a pathogen or parasite in my gut. The thought of a worm or a virus crawling around inside of me made me sick to my stomach. So, I dutifully took the antibiotics. After all, they were the "experts" and I was desperate to feel better. Some of the antibiotics were so strong that I had to lie on the floor because of the resulting nausea and fatigue. In the end, none of the treatments worked.

I did not improve, but I also didn't get much worse over the next few years. I learned to live with the bloating, the pain, and the embarrassment of frequently running to the bathroom. It put a serious crimp in my social life, but I had already run through a string of "experts" and nobody knew how to help me. So, I managed the hand I was dealt as best as I could.

Then, in about 2008, I took a turn for the worse. I was so bloated after every meal that I looked like I was five months pregnant. It was painful and nauseating. By this time I had earned my doctoral degree in Nutrition. Since I knew how the foods I ate were digested and assimilated into my body, I decided to become my own detective.

Fortunately, God blessed me with a fabulous husband right around this time. He became my co-detective. My husband is a chemical engineer so he brought a whole new perspective to the table. Together we scoured the scientific literature and taught each other what we learned. Then, one day, my husband stumbled upon a critical piece of information. He found a research article that mentioned leaky gut. At the time, not much was known about that condition. The words "leaky gut" were not commonly uttered in magazines or most Internet articles. We couldn't even find very much information about it in peer-reviewed journals. So, we came up with our own theory about what leaky gut was and how it applied to me specifically.

We theorized that **I had developed leaky gut from eating chemicals in my food** such as pesticides, herbicides, genetically modified organisms (GMOs), synthetic food additives, and gluten. All of these chemicals are abundant in our food supply, which we will discuss in section two of this book. For now, imagine your intestines lined with tiny gates. Those gates help determine which substances are allowed to travel from your intestines into the surrounding tissues and eventually into your blood stream. The foods we eat, along with the chemicals on those foods, can indirectly cause those gates to open really wide. When that happens, food, bacteria, and viral proteins can travel from your intestines into your blood stream where they do not belong. Your body, in turn, can see these substances as foreign invaders and attack them. This can lead to food allergies, food sensitivities, and even disease.[†] If our leaky gut theory was correct, we knew I needed to eat organic food and follow a gluten-free diet. However, the solution wouldn't be as simple as we thought.

We were lucky that God gave us a big clue up front: my gastrointestinal symptoms. I used to see my gut issue as a curse, but now I realize it was a blessing. It was the biggest clue we had that led us to the scene of the crime. For instance, we figured out that nearly every time I ate gluten, I experienced cramping. However, most people with gluten issues do not experience GI symptoms.[2] It's estimated that only one out of every seven people with gluten issues have GI symptoms.[2] That means roughly 14% of people who do have a problem with gluten will have GI symptoms. The remaining 86% of people with gluten issues may not show any symptoms until they are diagnosed with a diet-related disease such as diabetes, heart disease, autism, autoimmune disease, or ADHD.[2] There are over 200 medical conditions currently connected to gluten sensitivity, ranging from asthma to infertility.[3,4] I was blessed that my symptoms were obviously related to my gut.

Upon discovering the connection between diet and my gut, I immediately switched to organic and gluten-free foods. This was before gluten-free became a fad, so there weren't many gluten-free products on the market. I remember finding one store that sold a very small selection of roughly 10 items to pick from. I was elated! I bought boxes of gluten-free cereal, cookies, and noodles. There was only one flavor of each to choose from, but I didn't care. I had something to eat! Within a couple of days of eating gluten-free, I felt so much better. The cramping, bloating, and constipation were nearly gone. My husband and I rejoiced! We thought we solved the mystery that had baffled an entire team of medical experts for years. However, we quickly realized that even though I was doing better, my condition was not resolved.

After eating gluten-free for several weeks, I began to feel sick again. The cramping and bloating returned. It wasn't as bad as it had previously been, so we knew the gluten-free diet was helping. We were on the right track. But, over the next three years I had five miscarriages. I sought

---

† For additional information on the connection between the gut and disease, refer to *The Autoimmune Fix* by Dr. Tom O'Bryan.

help from a fertility expert who couldn't find anything wrong with me. I also developed a tumor on the white of my eye (sclera). According to the ophthalmologist, the cause was unknown and the tumor would eventually cover my cornea, effectively blinding me.

The experts didn't have any answers and I didn't know where to look next, but I knew all of my symptoms had to be connected to my diet. So, I started a strict diet elimination-reintroduction protocol. This took quite some time because my reaction to certain foods would linger for weeks, namely the constipation. And, to truly evaluate each food item, I needed a strong and repeatable baseline.

After about two years of subjecting myself to my own dietary study, I had successfully created a list of "do not eat" foods. The list was long and included basic staples like beans, milk, rice, corn, oats, all gluten, certain nuts, soy, and meat. Eating became very difficult. My options were limited. Plus, I was making all of my food from scratch because all canned and processed foods made me sick. Even gluten-free processed foods were making me sick at this point. Consequently, my food list became my lifeline. It wasn't complete, but I knew that we were close because as long as I stuck with my list I felt the best I had in nearly 20 years. My bloating had reduced and my energy level had increased.

Since I was beginning to feel better, my husband and I turned our efforts towards finding any common threads between the foods on my list. For instance, what do rice and corn have in common? Are they metabolized differently in the body? It wasn't enough to know which foods to eliminate from my diet. I needed to know what damage, if any, these foods had caused my body so that I could correct it and be completely healed. To do that, I needed to know how it all connected.

We spent weeks trying to connect the dots, with no success. During that time, my body began to reject nearly all foods, even foods that were on my "okay to eat" list. These were simple foods like apples and bananas. How could my body react to a banana? I became so frustrated that I tried a different dietary approach. I decided to try the GAPS diet, a gut healing diet. I knew that all my health issues stemmed from leaky gut and if I could heal my gut then perhaps I could eat a greater variety of food.

I learned how to make bone broths and meat stock, both staples on the GAPS diet. I took out all dairy and nuts. I essentially ate cooked vegetables, soup, and broths. I still couldn't eat meat. My body rejected it. So I drank the broth and stock, which was like eating a bowl of liquid fat. The thought grossed me out but, surprisingly, my body loved the fat. I suddenly had more energy. I was finally able to cook a full meal without having to sit down to take a break! I still couldn't walk up the stairs without getting winded, or chase my kids around the house, but it was an improvement none-the-less. And, as long as I stayed on the strict GAPS diet, my bloating went down. It wasn't gone, but it had improved.

A couple months later, while still on the GAPS diet, I took a turn for the worse. More foods turned against me. So, I figured my gut was not healed yet. I had previously been diagnosed with a yeast overgrowth, which I knew could cause leaky gut. At the time of my diagnosis I was pregnant, so I declined treatment. But, now that my son had been born, I decided to try the candida diet. That meant eliminating almost all sugar from my diet, even carrots and peas. That was hard! I combined a candida diet with the use of essential oils. It worked perfectly!

In the first week of the candida diet, I experienced nearly every sugar withdrawal symptom imaginable. I even got hives for the first time in my life. It was awful. I was tired, irritated, bloated, nauseated, restless, and simply annoyed. However, the more withdrawal symptoms I experienced, the stronger my dedication became. My body's response to a very low-sugar diet confirmed that I was hooked on sugar and that I had too much yeast. I could actually see yeast cultures when I used the bathroom. I diligently stuck to my very low-sugar diet for over two months. The deprivation was worth it because my next yeast overgrowth test came back negative.

However, my GI symptoms did not improve. I still could not eat any new foods, the bloating returned, and my energy level was declining quickly. In addition, my body began to reject the bone broth and meat stock. Plus, a new symptom appeared: low-grade muscle pain throughout my body. The pain was constant, but it moved to different parts of my body. Much to my disappointment, I had to face reality. No matter what dietary treatment I tried, I was getting worse and I was running out of leads. I didn't know where to turn next.

Soon after, I learned about free online health summits that feature experts in disease and diet. I spent the next one-and-a-half years listening to these health summits nearly every single week. Some weeks I'd listen for 30-40 hours. I was desperate for an answer and determined to never give up.

One day, while listening to a talk by Dr. Tom O'Bryan, author of *The Autoimmune Fix,* I pieced together a big part of the puzzle. I learned that the common thread in most all of the foods on my list was gluten.[2] I did not know that rice and corn contained a compound that looks like gluten. That meant I was still eating gluten without knowing it. It also meant that all the gluten-free products I had eaten over the past several years actually contained gluten, or gluten-like compounds! That's why I got better on the gluten-free diet but then got worse again. My body got a break from eating wheat and I felt better, but then the rice and corn started punching holes in my gut and so I got worse.

I was elated to find that answer, but I was also confused. The gluten-free products I bought in the store contained rice and corn, but they were labeled as gluten-free. If rice and corn contain gluten, then why are they labeled as gluten-free?

I did some digging. It didn't take long to find out that the "mislabeling" of these foods was because of the FDA. The FDA is in charge of food labels. Consequently, they decide what is considered gluten-free. In making that determination, the FDA used an outdated definition of gluten that dates back to the early 1930s. At that time, a pediatrician from the Netherlands linked wheat to Celiac Disease. Then, during the 1944 "Winter of Starvation," he observed improvements in his patients symptoms during a wheat shortage.[5] Consequently, he began testing other foods on his patients, including rye. These were food staples in that country, at that time, so naturally he characterized gluten-containing foods based on what the people were readily eating.[5]

Now we know there are over 2,000 gluten compounds.[2] But, the FDA does not acknowledge this new information. Instead, they base our food labels on outdated and inaccurate information, which puts some of us directly in harm's way. Take me, for example. I learned in the health summit that every time I ate gluten, including rice and corn, it made me sick. It contributed to my leaky gut.

Consequently, I removed all known gluten compounds from my diet, including corn and rice. But, after a couple of months on this new diet, I still had the muscular pain and fatigue. In fact, I felt worse. For much of the day I resorted to lying on the floor because the pain was so intense. I didn't allow myself to take anti-inflammatories because I knew that while they would provide relief in the moment, they could actually harm my gut. So, I dealt with the pain as best as I knew how.

Then, in 2016, my entire family got the flu. But, I was the only one who ended up in the emergency room. My blood pressure dropped very low. I became dehydrated, and was unable to stand. That was the straw that broke the camel's back, so to speak. From that moment on, my health began to rapidly decline.

Over the next month, I lost more than ten pounds. It wasn't the good type of weight loss where you are thrilled to be achieving your New Year's resolution. Quite the contrary, for the first time in my 20 years of illness, I had begun the process of **muscle wasting.** It's similar to what cancer patients can experience. And, I couldn't stop it. No matter how much I ate, I kept losing weight. For the first time in 20 years of dealing with my illness, I was scared for my life.

I used to be a competitive athlete who cycled over 100 miles a week and hiked on the weekend, and now I was reduced to lying on the floor because sitting was too difficult. The muscle pain and fatigue were overwhelming. It became difficult to even wrap my hand around a cup, or stand long enough to wash the dishes after lunch. In addition, a new symptom appeared: **my gums began to ache**. I felt like my teeth were beginning to loosen. It hurt every time I chewed. And, at times, it became **difficult to breathe**.

I didn't know what to do. I had already eliminated every trigger from my diet that I could think of. The list of foods I could eat had dwindled to half a sheet of paper. And now, once again, foods that I could previously eat were added to my "do not eat" list. I was in a downward spiral with no parachute to be found. So, I got down on my knees and prayed. For the first time in my life, I surrendered to God.

God not only gave me a parachute, He opened it for me. The very next week, while listening to a fabulous health summit about food and disease, my prayers were answered. I listened to every lecture in that 40 hour summit. One expert stood out: Dr. Osborne. As soon as I heard his voice, I knew I was meant to call him. It was strange because I had listened to summits for nearly two years and never had this type of response before. In addition, his practice is based out of Texas and he's world-renowned for his work in helping people like me. So, the odds of getting in to see him were not high. Plus, he was about to release a book titled, *No Grain, No Pain,* so I knew he would be in greater demand than ever. Still, that voice inside of me was confident that he was the missing piece to the puzzle. With his help, I knew we would solve my mystery once and for all.

My husband came home from work that night and, after getting the kids to bed, I told him that I knew I needed the kind of help that insurance wouldn't cover and that we both knew would be very expensive. My medical bills had already been piling up for years so I knew he would not be thrilled at my new revelation. I choked back my tears as I told him that I knew if I didn't get help, I would not live to see our children grow up. I knew that if I continued on my current path, I would not live to see them graduate, get married, or have children. I didn't know what was wrong with me, but I knew the seriousness of muscle wasting. I could literally picture what was happening inside of me. Even though I was eating almost constantly, **my body was literally starving to death.** And, I couldn't stop it.

I didn't want to live my life in pain any more. I longed to have enough energy and strength to chase my children around the house, to play ball with them outside, to teach them how to ride a bike, and to simply sit on the grass at the park while enjoying a picnic lunch together without having to lay down. I wanted my life back.

My husband listened to every word I spoke and felt every tear I cried. When I was finished, he only asked one question: "Do you think this guy can help you?" I immediately replied, "Yes." A simple yes is all it took. His support gave me the freedom to do what was long overdue: To decide.

I made a choice that night. I decided I'd had enough. Life was too good to not exhaust every avenue possible for even the minuscule chance that I could be healed, no matter how much it cost. I decided I was worth it. **That was my turning point.**

I called Dr. Osborne's office the next morning. That phone call changed my life.

Dr. Osborne figured out the remaining foods that were making me sick. Most of the triggers I had already identified through my diet elimination-reintroduction protocol, but there were some surprises that popped up, like bay leaf. I would never have guessed that a seasoning was making me sick.

I also tested **positive for arsenic poisoning**, which I believe came from eating so much rice in the form of processed gluten-free products. Did you know that even organic rice can be contaminated with arsenic?[6] Arsenic can cause cancer, heart disease and diabetes.[6] As bad as that sounds, arsenic poisoning was not my biggest problem.

I was **deficient in 15 nutrients**! Even though I consumed these nutrients on a regular basis in the form of supplements, my body could not properly absorb them because the lining of my gut was so damaged from eating chemicals in our food supply. Consequently, my health had deteriorated so dramatically that I was **diagnosed as borderline for both beriberi and pellagra**. These aren't diseases we typically see in the United States any more. Both of these diseases are caused by nutrient deficiencies, both **can lead to death**, and both were almost entirely eradicated in the early to mid-1900s.[7] Pellagra can also result in dementia and has become so rare that it mainly occurs in refugees and during times of emergency in developing countries.[7] Beriberi can lead to heart failure and muscle paralysis, and most commonly occurs in alcoholics.[8] Since I don't live in a third world country and I don't drink alcohol, the diagnosis was shocking. But, it wasn't as upsetting as what came next.

Dr. Osborne diagnosed me with an active autoimmune disease. Genetics played a role, but **my autoimmune disease largely developed from eating food**! That's how powerful food can be. I developed leaky gut from eating food, along with the chemicals on the food. Consequently, my immune system was on high alert all the time. Not only was my body attacking all glutens that I ate, my body had been fighting this losing battle for so long that it had begun attacking itself. That's why I had pain through my body.

It's also why I developed muscle wasting. In a nutshell, **my body was ripping apart my muscles** and other tissues to make the antibodies it needed to attack itself. I didn't know it at the time, but I was experiencing an *advanced stage* of an active Autoimmune Disease. My immune system became so hyperactive that I began developing allergies to foods like almonds. I also developed adverse reactions to chemicals like the dyes in my sheets and my husband's mouthwash. So, what was the solution?

I eliminated the remaining foods from my diet that were triggering an immune response, supplemented with the right nutrients for my body, balanced my gut microflora, and changed my lifestyle.[‡] After only 8 months, I'm now mostly pain-free! And, I have enough energy to keep up with my children, including chasing them around the house playing foam dart gun wars. I even accomplished a life-long dream of running

---

‡ For additional information on the connection between pain and diet, particularly grain, please refer to *No Grain, No Pain* by Dr. Peter Osborne.

up the 72 "Rocky steps" of the Philadelphia Art Museum that were featured in the movie *Rocky*!

Sadly, what happened to me is all too common in America today. No matter how you look at the situation, **our families are getting sicker.** Half of all Americans currently suffer from at least one chronic illness such as heart disease, cancer, or diabetes.[9] In addition, one in three adults are obese.[9] These chronic diseases can shorten your life span. For instance, diabetics live roughly 13 years less than non-diabetics while obesity can reduce your lifespan by 5 to 20 years.[10]

Of all the chronic diseases, the leading killer in the United States is heart disease, which is responsible for one in every four deaths.[11] Every minute, someone dies in America from an issue related to heart disease, such as a heart attack.[11] As bad as that sounds, it's only getting worse. Chronic disease is currently increasing at a steady rate across all age groups.[12,13] The Center for Disease Control predicts that by 2020 nearly two million Americans will be diagnosed with cancer every year, which would make cancer the leading cause of death in America.[14]

Even children are sicker. The number of chronic illnesses among children in America has quadrupled since the 1960s.[15] Currently, more than 25% of children suffer from a chronic disease and that number is expected to rise.[12] In addition, 60% of children between the ages of five and ten years old already have at least one risk factor for heart disease, while more than 20% of children have two or more risk factors.[15,16] What does this mean for our children? For the first time in the history of the United States, children may live shorter lives than their parents.[10,13]

But, we don't need statistics to tell us that children are getting sicker. Have you noticed how many children have food allergies these days? I can't go to a school, daycare, or Sunday school class without seeing an allergy alert posted on the classroom door! Everyone I know has at least one family member who currently suffers from an allergy or a gut-related illness. Why? Why are we getting sicker?

**Our food system is not designed to protect our long-term health.**

My illness wasn't instantaneous. It didn't just appear after eating at my favorite hamburger joint. It happened over 20 years. I ate the chemicals that are prevalent in our food supply without any noticeable effects for half of my life. I went through life thinking I was fine, feeling invincible, and then I slowly became debilitatingly ill.

The increase we see in chronic diseases among both adults and children is most likely due to a combination of factors, including: more time on electronics and less time playing outdoors and exercising, more chemicals in our environment, and possibly more exposure to radiation through cell phones and other hand-held electronic devices, just to name a few. Is it possible that diet has contributed to the increase in disease we are seeing in America?

Yes!

**Our food supply has been linked with a whole slew of Western diseases** such as heart disease, diabetes, cancer, and arthritis.[17–21] In fact, an article published in *The American Journal of Clinical Nutrition* in 2005 concluded that while genetics and the environment play a role, "…evidence gleaned over the past 3 decades now indicates that virtually all so-called diseases of civilization have multifactorial dietary elements that underlie their etiology."[20]

That makes sense because as Americans have gotten sicker within the past 60 years, our food has undergone major changes:[19–23]

- The introduction of synthetic pesticides and herbicides occurred just before this time period.[24] And, the amount of chemicals sprayed on our food crops has increased dramatically over the past 60 years.[25–28] For instance, according to the USDA, roughly 5-10% of corn crops were treated with herbicides in 1952.[29] By 1980, herbicides were sprayed on 90-99% of corn crops.[29] That's bad news for us since glyphosate, the most widely used herbicide today, was declared by the World Health Organization to be "probably carcinogenic to humans."[30]
- In addition, the consumption of synthetic chemical additives has also increased as our diets have shifted further away from whole foods and predominately towards processed foods.[31]
- GMOs appeared on the scene during this time period as well.[32] They *fundamentally* transformed our food supply.

We will discuss all of that in more detail in section two of this book. But, before we dive into the corruption that exists in our food supply, I need to confess that I was embarrassed, for a long time, to admit that I got debilitatingly ill from eating food. How did someone with my knowledge of food end up with an autoimmune disease, arsenic poisoning, and deficiencies in 15 nutrients? Shouldn't I have known better?

The answer is simple, actually. I didn't know what's in our food.

I thought I knew a lot about food. I have a degree hanging on my wall that tells me I know a lot about food. I've studied food for over half my life. I can tell you what happens inside your body when you eat any food, such as a hamburger. I can trace every detailed chemical reaction that occurs from the time that piece of meat enters your mouth until it leaves your body. But, what good was that knowledge when I was lying on the floor in tears because I didn't have the strength or energy to play with my baby boy? I couldn't fix my own diet-induced problem. I couldn't help myself. Why?

I had a veil of trust covering my eyes, an unearned veil.

# CHAPTER 2:

# THE VEIL

I t's as though I've worn a veil over my eyes my whole life, blinding me from the truth about what's really in our food. My veil looked like this:

Food companies work hard to provide us with the best-tasting food possible, using the latest technology available, at a cost you and I can afford. They fortify our foods with vitamins and minerals to ensure we get enough nutrients every day.

"Experts" help the food companies. Researchers at the most prestigious universities throughout the United States are constantly pushing the boundaries of science to give us the healthiest and best-tasting food possible. They work with medical associations, like the American Heart Association, and other scientific groups to determine which nutrients will help prevent us from getting diseases. Then, they invent ways to pack our favorite foods full of these healthy nutrients, like adding vitamin D to our milk. They even invent new flavors so we have something to look forward to.

Government has the most important job of all. They make sure all of our food is safe to eat. They hire the best scientists, who routinely test our food for safety and provide stringent guidelines that all food companies must follow. Our government works hard to keep the food companies in check through regulations, laws, and inspections. All the food in our grocery stores has been inspected and approved by our government. They also create our dietary guidelines, including the food pyramid, so that Americans know exactly what they should eat to be as healthy as possible.

If that's roughly your view of our food supply, you're not alone. That's the veil of unearned trust. I had one. How do you know if you have a veil of unearned trust?

Here are a few examples to help you determine if you have a veil, even just a partial one:

- If you shop at your local grocery store and never question the safety of the food.
- If you think your food is safe because it's organic.
- If you think the FDA conducts safety tests on our food.
- If you assume that *someone* is making sure your food is safe to eat.
- If you take dietary advice from your doctor because you think doctors are well trained in nutrition.
- If you think eating red meat causes heart disease.
- If you think eating saturated fat causes heart disease.
- If you don't read the ingredient label before you eat a food.
- If you read the ingredient label, see a word you cannot pronounce, and you eat the food anyway.
- If you read the ingredient label, but only for the fat content.
- If you put more thought into the flavor than the ingredients.
- If you shop for food by looking for the cheapest brand.
- If you think low-fat means it won't make you fat.
- If you think low-fat is healthier than whole-fat.
- If you think wheat bread is simply a flavor of bread, like sour dough or French (my husband thought this was true until he was 28 years old).
- If you think the processed foods we love, like frozen pizzas and mini-donuts, are created by professional chefs in a kitchen.

I didn't even realize I had a veil until I got debilitating sick from our food. I am not suggesting that diet is the only factor involved in the rise in diseases we are experiencing in America. But, diet is one key player. Clearly, **as our food supply has changed, Americans have gotten sicker.** And, the most susceptible populations are babies and children because of their smaller body weight, higher cell turn over, decreased ability to eliminate certain chemicals from the body, and larger surface-to-volume area of the skin, particularly in babies.[1,2] Yet, many of us don't seem to be disturbed by the chemicals that are lurking in our foods. We buy chemically laced foods and we feed them to our families. Why?

People may not realize that eating chemicals in low doses can affect their health over time. You may be able to eat the chemicals in our food supply for 10, 20, or even 30 years with little to no noticeable consequence, leading you to believe the food is okay to eat. Then, 40 years down the road, you're diagnosed with cancer, an autoimmune condition, or diabetes, and you wonder how it happened.

Medical doctors will theorize about why you got sick. They might tell you it's genetic or that you don't exercise enough. They don't typically connect the origin of your disease to diet, but we shouldn't expect them to. Many doctors don't receive adequate nutrition training in school. Roughly two-thirds of medical schools in the United States don't require doctors to take a single class on nutrition.[3] Yet, many of us rely on medical doctors for diet advice. Regardless, doctors usually prescribe diet changes when someone is diagnosed with a chronic or inflammatory disease. That means our medical establishment does recognize that diet plays a role in all of those diseases.

Yet, many of us don't act on that knowledge. We invest time, money, and energy into our long-term health in other areas of our lives, including check-ups at our doctor's office and expensive gym memberships. But, when it comes to the food we eat, we largely dismiss the potential long-term health consequences of our choices. That's the veil of unearned trust in action, and it comes with consequences. It wasn't until I got sick that I understood the consequence of my veil.

Let me be clear, this book is not about convincing you that synthetic chemicals are bad or that you shouldn't eat genetically modified organisms (GMOs), even though you may come to these conclusions on your own. Those are individual decisions that only you can decide for yourself. This book reveals the truth behind what's in our food, how it got there, who's responsible, and how we can fix it. Here's a glimpse into the reality of the situation we face:

- Large food companies spend billions of dollars every year lobbying Congress and making backdoor deals.[4] Congress, in turn, passes laws that carve out exceptions and loopholes in favor of large food companies, while squeezing out your local farmer and small business owner.[4] For example, politicians largely decide what's on your dinner plate by picking which crops are winners and losers. In the end, we lose. We'll discuss this in chapter five.

- Meanwhile, the FDA claims to oversee the safety of our food but they look the other way when synthetic chemicals that have not been tested for safety are added to our cookies, cakes and breads.[5] In addition, we are being used as un-consenting guinea pigs for companies who want to test out their latest laboratory creations. For example, GMOs are now abundant in our processed foods.[6,7] Most of us eat them every day and don't even know it because they aren't labeled. That's a problem because GMOs have never been adequately tested for long-term safety.[8] Nobody knows what effect they will have on our long-term health. The FDA knows this is happening and, as I'll reveal in section two of this book, they sanctioned it. So much for "protecting and promoting" our health, as the FDAs tagline touts.[9]

- Additionally, some scientists are resorting to falsifying and manipulating data.[10] Why? The heavy demand to obtain a steady flow of grant money has turned our great-thinkers into mercenaries. Industry is happy to fill their pockets with grant money, as long as the results from their research studies favor the company.[11] And we wonder why there is so much conflicting information in the news about nutrition: One day scientists claim a food is good for us and the next day it's on their black list. The days of independent research are over. Welcome to the new era of researchers for hire.

All of that is bad, really bad, and it is just the tip of the iceberg. As you can glean from these examples, we are not only losing our health, our freedom is eroding. We'll discuss the loss of our freedom throughout this book as I reveal more truths about our food supply. But, for now let's honestly ask ourselves: What's the *real problem* with our food supply? Who's ultimately responsible for this mess?

CHAPTER 3:

# THE ROOT OF THE PROBLEM

**"We the People" are the root of the problem.**

We created this situation. We are the real problem. Allow me to explain.

I love birthday parties! My girlfriend hosts the best birthday parties for her children. She has the most creative decorations, the best games, and the cutest cupcakes. Her cupcakes steal the show every year. The cake portion is brilliantly colored in blues, greens, and reds. The frosting is rainbow colored with fun-shaped sprinkles on top. And, every year the same thing happens: My girlfriends contemplate if they should eat a cupcake because they are high in calories. Those of us with children wonder if we should give them a whole cupcake or just a half because they are high in sugar. And, I always eat two cupcakes myself!

They were made from packaged mixes that feature neon-colored cupcakes with vibrantly colored confetti-like sprinkles on top. Have you seen them on your grocery store shelf? It's the type of advertising that your child sees and immediately asks if he can have it. You might be tempted to buy it because you want your kids to be happy and because these foods are easy to make and are cheaper than the healthier alternatives. Why wouldn't you buy it?

I used to buy those cupcake mixes. Then I flipped over the box and read the ingredient label. I quickly realized why I would never buy them again. There were multiple cupcake flavors, or should I say "colorings," to choose from including:[1]

- "Neon Yellow," which contained Yellow 5
- "Bold Purple," which contained Blue 1 and Red 40
- "Aqua Blue," which contained Blue 1
- "Orange Allstar," which contained Yellow 6
- "Radiant Red," which contained Red 40
- "Vibrant Green," which contained Yellow 5 and Blue 1

Each cupcake mix contained dyes, some of which are linked to cancer, hyperactivity, loss of mental focus, and allergic reactions.[2–7] In addition to dyes, those cupcake mixes contained propylene glycol and BHT (butylated hydroxytoulene). Propylene glycol is used to make antifreeze and paint.[8] It may be toxic to the central nervous system.[9] BHT is used in embalming fluid and jet fuel.[8] It has been shown in studies to promote tumor growth and damage DNA.[6,10–12]

The frosting was even worse. It contained seven dyes, including Red 40, which has been linked to allergic reactions and tumor promotion, and it may contain cancer-causing contaminants.[2,6,7,13] The frosting also contained genetically modified corn and soy, wax, and polysorbate 60. Polysorbate 60 is made from petroleum, which is oil.[14] How did cancer-causing dyes and paint chemicals get into our cupcakes? Who let this happen?

We did.

Many of us unknowingly celebrate our child's life by giving them foods that can hurt them, specifically in the long-term. I'm as guilty as anyone. I not only fed those cupcakes to my children at my friends' house, I made them for my own child's birthday parties. My friends and I simply weren't aware of the potential dangers that lurk in our food. We assumed the cupcakes must be safe because they are sold in our supermarkets. Somebody must be testing them for safety, right? Besides, we eat these foods and we seem okay right now. So, how bad could they really be?

That's the veil of unearned trust.
And, that veil comes with consequences.

In our birthday example, wearing the veil meant that what should have been a care-free, fun-filled birthday celebration turned into a day where our children feasted on treats containing chemicals that may cause cancer. Does that mean my friends and I are bad moms?

No, of course not. We don't intentionally feed our children foods that will harm them. But, it does mean that we were part of the problem: Not because we chose to feed our children potentially harmful chemicals. That's an individual choice. We were part of the problem because we fed our families those cupcakes without knowing what's in them, and without considering the potential consequences of our decision. We were uninformed consumers.

That may sound harsh, but we have to face the reality of the situation if we are going to fix it. Trust me, I didn't know what's really in our food for most of my life, and look where it got me: suffering from arsenic poisoning and a food-induced disease. I was part of the problem.

**Are you part of the problem?**

Whether you realize it or not, you are already voicing your opinion about our food supply: **You speak with your dollars**. Each time you spend your money at a grocery store, fast food restaurant, vending machine, or hot dog stand, you are speaking with your dollars. Every day, the food industry and the government hear your message loud and clear. For instance, if you buy the neon-colored cupcake mixes, you are telling our government and the company who made that product that you are okay with eating dyes that may cause cancer, you are okay with eating chemicals that are found in antifreeze, and you are okay with eating chemicals that might damage your DNA. When you drink Mountain Dew®, you are telling PepsiCo, Inc. (The maker of Mountain Dew®) and the FDA that you are okay with drinking flame-retardants.[15] And, when you buy genetically modified foods, you are saying you think it's okay for "experts" to change the unique genetic make-up of our plants and animals.

**Our food supply is a reflection of how we spend our dollars.** Consequently, it changes with the choices we make on a daily basis. That's fabulous news because it means we can begin to change our food supply right now! The beauty of the free market is that we can change how we spend our money and the market will adapt. With each purchase, we have the ability to shape our food supply into what we want it to be.

Let me give you an example of how your dollars, in other words your decisions, helped create our current food supply and how your dollars can change it. I grew up eating Doritos®. The maker of Doritos®, Frito-Lay North America, Inc., creates their nacho cheese flavored chip using Red 40, an artificial coloring that can damage DNA and promote tumor growth in mice, as well as hyperactivity in children.[2,6,13,16] In addition, these tasty chips provide you with a daily helping of disodium inosinate, which has been suspected of damaging organs, including effecting fertility.[16,17] The chips also contain monosodium glutamate, which is an excitatory neurotransmitter that can damage and even kill cells, including brain cells.[18–25] It has also reportedly caused headaches, weakness, rapid heartbeat, inability to focus, and diarrhea.[24] Why are these chemicals in our Doritos®?

Because of us!

We buy Doritos® regardless of the chemicals they contain. The ingredients are listed on the package. It's our responsibility to read the ingredient label and decide for ourselves if we want to eat that product. In regards to Doritos®, the marketplace has spoken. Since we continue to buy these chips, Frito-Lay North America, Inc. continues to put dyes and other synthetic chemicals in our Doritos®. Instead of adding monosodium glutamate to Doritos®, Frito-Lay North America, Inc. could have chosen a more natural ingredient such as rosemary extract.[26,27] A large manufacturing company in the United Kingdom has already done this.[26] So, why are Doritos® made with monosodium glutamate instead of rosemary extract?

It's cheap and Americans are willing to eat it.

Let's assume we didn't want to eat monosodium glutamate in our chips. Using the market-based food system, how could we get Frito-Lay North America, Inc. to stop putting monosodium glutamate in our Doritos®?

It's simple: stop buying them.

**Business responds to consumer demand.** If we voiced our concern, Frito-Lay North America, Inc. would stop using monosodium glutamate. But, we already know this, at least on some level. Many of us already exercise our power as consumers. For instance, when Americans found out that Doritos® contained hydrogenated oils, the people rose up.[28,29] Consumers demanded that Frito-Lay North America, Inc. remove trans fats from their Doritos® and the company responded to their demand.[28] Consequently, since 2003, Doritos® no longer contain trans fats.[30] **When we are informed consumers, the market-based solution can work.**

We have the power to create the food supply we desire. To harness that power, we need to be aware of what's in our food and learn how to use our power as consumers. If we don't consciously place demand on companies, we end up suppressing our voice, along with our power. We lose freedom.

**This book is designed to help you harness your power as a consumer by revealing what's in your food and providing options for how you can reclaim your voice.**

As you learn the truth about our food supply, the information can be upsetting and overwhelming. Please keep in mind, there is a solution. Abraham Lincoln said that our government is, "of the people, by the people, for the people."[31] That holds true for our food supply as well. If we don't like the current system, it's up to us to change it.

I am the solution.
**You are the solution.**
"We the People" are the solution.

We can fix this problem by moving the market: Easy solutions are provided at the end of each chapter in section two. In addition, section three focuses solely on solutions. And, a free companion guide containing suggestions on how to move the market is available at www.handsoffmyfood.com.

As you will see during our time together, government and industry are not the solution. For instance, let's assume we wanted to remove the potentially harmful chemicals from Doritos®. Some people would call on government to create more laws and regulations that would force Frito-Lay North America, Inc. to remove the chemicals. That might initially sound like a good idea, but relinquishing our authority to the government adds to the problem. That solution grows government, which thickens our veil of unearned trust. As we hand more responsibility and authority to the FDA and USDA, they get larger and more laws are enacted. Consequently, people feel safer. People believe the government is watching over their food supply. They believe the government is forcing these companies to remove potentially harmful chemicals from our favorite treats. But, is that really the case?

I used to think the FDA conducted stringent tests on chemicals before deciding which ones could be added to our food. It's a logical assumption. After all, the FDA requires years of testing before pharmaceutical drugs are released on the market, so it's logical to assume that our food is tested as well. But, that's simply not true. The FDA does not conduct safety tests on chemicals added to our foods. Instead, **the FDA relies on companies to determine the safety of their own chemicals.**[32–34]

In our Doritos® example, monosodium glutamate is "generally recognized as safe" (GRAS). That means it's a chemical that the government does not test for safety, does not regulate, and does not approve for use in our food.[32] Instead, the safety and regulation of the chemical is the responsibility of the company. Frito-Lay North America, Inc. can decide that monosodium glutamate is safe by hiring a scientific "expert" to write a letter declaring it to be safe. These "experts" are frequently bought and paid for by industry. They are employees or consultants, or sometimes they own stock in the company.[32,35] Although the actions of these "experts" may be morally questionable, they are not the real problem. They are responding to the system that has been created by us.

In our Doritos® example, the misleading role of government is evident. The FDA claims to "promote and protect your health," but they don't weigh in on the chemicals added to our foods that are GRAS. Because they don't declare the ingredients in Doritos® to either be "bad" or "safe" for you to eat, the perception is that these ingredients are safe. The consumer sees Doritos® on the supermarket shelf and might assume the FDA approved them for us to eat, even though the FDA does not see it that way.

The FDA is very clear that they do not approve or disapprove of the ingredients in Doritos®. They clearly acknowledge that the company is responsible for determining the safety of their own product.[36] Thus, our recourse is to sue the company if we get sick from their food. However, since there are over 10,000 chemical additives in our food supply, and you may not present with a disease until years down the road, you cannot prove liability.[32] In essence, the company is not held responsible or accountable. So much for the government being the watchdog that they claim to be!

The government also promotes Doritos® by subsidizing several ingredients contained within the chips, including corn, corn oil, maltodextrin, and corn flour.[37–39] In other words, the government uses our tax dollars to help make those ingredients cheaper, which incentivizes companies to choose those ingredients when making our food. That's bad news for us because those foods are making us sick, according to a study conducted by the Centers for Disease Control.[40,41]

Government can't fix the problem. In our Doritos® example, the government played a key role in getting those potentially harmful chemicals into our food. They also provided consumers with a false sense of security by declaring to be our watchdog, but really abdicating their perceived responsibility to the company. Government made the problem worse.

While government is not the solution, it's not the real problem either. Government only grows as big as the people allow it to get. The bigger it gets, the more loopholes exist and the more mistakes are made. Government is made up of people, and people are fallible. Blaming the government for our problems is like blaming ourselves because we allowed it to grow and to expand its authority over our lives. Besides, as I previously mentioned, the more the government intervenes with our daily lives, the thicker our veil becomes. **Government perpetuates the veil of unearned trust.**

Industry is not the solution either, but it is also not the real problem. Businesses respond to incentives. As government grows in size and influence, an environment ensues where it is treated like a money piñata. For instance, when government grows large enough, it is in the best interest of a company to lobby Congress to pass laws that favor their business. This is the natural evolution of a company based on the circumstances that large government creates. Perhaps it would help to think of corporations as living entities. In 2010, the Supreme Court declared corporations to be people.[42,43] Just like a human adapts to their environment, so does a corporation. It will adapt to maximize its potential or reproductive ability, which is measured by its profits. Hence, when an opportunity for increased profits arises, such as loopholes that allow companies to add chemicals to our foods without going through government "red tape" or the passing of legislature that decreases the cost of ingredients, it is natural for the company to seize the opportunity.

Let me give you a real-life example. When I worked for a large supplement company, they supported more government regulation. Why would any company want more government "red tape"? It was a way to crush their smaller competitors. It costs money to get through government "red tape". Consequently, it's more difficult for a smaller company to keep up with the cost of business when more government regulations are imposed. It's a brilliant strategy; morally questionable, but brilliant. The larger company adapted to the environment that big government created by finding their evolutionary advantage. Therefore, business is not the real problem. It is a reflection of the environment we have created.

Isn't it ultimately the fault of Frito-Lay North America, Inc. that potentially harmful chemicals are in our chips? After all, they added the synthetic chemicals to our chips in the first place. If a company were practicing conscious capitalism then they would choose natural ingredients instead of untested, synthetic chemicals and artificial dyes, right? They would conduct long-term studies on these chemicals to make sure they are safe, right?

Wrong.

Remember, companies are "people." And, like people, they often work on greed and laziness. Additionally, just like us, they require incentives. Have *we* given them an incentive to ensure our food is safe?

Yes, in terms of short-term illness we do provide the necessary incentive to companies. We've done a great job with ensuring our food supply is safe in the short-term, as evidenced by the Chipotle® example. But, what part have we played in ensuring our *long-term* health? Have we incentivized industry to conduct long-term safety testing on the chemicals they put in our foods?

Let's look at our Doritos® example. Have we incentivized Frito-Lay North America, Inc. to safety test the chemicals in our Doritos®?

No.

How do I know? Doritos® remain the best-selling chip worldwide.[44,45]

To change our food supply, we need to provide companies with incentives. To do that, we must be informed consumers. What would happen if we became a more informed citizenry?

All we have to do is look at Europe to see the possibility. When Europeans found out that companies were adding GMOs to their food supply, the people rose up against it.[46] Consequently, they moved the market.

Companies like Pepsi-Cola®, Heinz®, Mars®, and Kellogg's® responded to consumer demand by removing GMO ingredients from the foods they sell in Europe. McDonald's® even removed GMOs from their menus in Europe. However, they still add GMOs to our food in America.[47] Why?

We never demanded that GMOs be removed from our food. Instead, we consented to GMOs through our willingness to eat them. Consequently, most of us eat GMOs every day and don't even know it. In fact, you eat them in your Doritos®.

So, what are Americans demanding? Let's take a moment and be completely honest. Ask yourself: **How am I speaking with my dollars?**

- What message am I sending to the food industry?
- What message am I sending to our government?
- Am I supporting companies that are aligned with my values and principles?

I'm not giving industry, government, or "experts" a free pass or excusing their actions. Clearly, they all have a hand in this mess we call our food supply, which we will discuss throughout this book. However, the responsibility for our food falls on our shoulders. And we've stopped protecting our food. Instead, we rely on the government and the food industry to protect it for us. Consequently, our food is more adulterated today than ever before in the history of our Nation. In addition, we are less free today because we've relinquished our authority over our food.

We'll discuss all of that in section two. But, for now, let's go back to where it all began. When did the veil fall over the eyes of Americans? When did we abdicate our responsibility for our own food?

# CHAPTER 4:

# BIRTH OF THE VEIL

"The thing that bugs me is that people think the FDA is protecting them. It isn't. What the FDA is doing and what the public think it's doing are as different as night and day."[1]

—*Herbert Lay,* **Former FDA Commissioner**

Our food is more dangerous than it has ever been in the history of our nation, and it's largely because of our veil of unearned trust. That veil began to fall over the eyes of Americans with the birth of the Food and Drug Administration (FDA). With the passage of just two laws, control over our food supply was *permanently* changed. On that historic day in 1906, the federal government placed a firm grip on our food supply. It has been tightening that grip ever since. But, it didn't come easy. The road to centralization of our food supply was paved with many roadblocks. It would take a "poison squad," a book that hit us in the stomach, and a Progressive president before this revolutionary new era of food regulation took hold of America and slowly strangled her.

## Happy Birthday, FDA!

The FDA declares itself to be "the oldest comprehensive consumer protection agency in the U.S. federal government."[2] According to their website, the FDA is responsible for "Protecting the public health by assuring that foods are safe, wholesome, sanitary and properly labeled."[2] They oversee 80% of our food supply. The USDA has authority over the remaining 20%, including meat from livestock, poultry, and some egg products.[3] How did the FDA acquire so much authority over our food supply? To answer that question, we should take a step back and ask: Why do we have the FDA? The FDA did not exist at the birth of our nation. So, when did we get the FDA and why?

The FDA was given its official name in 1930; however, its birthday is much earlier. The seeds of the organization were planted in 1862. That was the year the U.S. Department of Agriculture was created. America was in the midst of the Civil War and the country needed more food. So, the USDA was created to help supply the army with food.[2,4]

It didn't take long for the roots of government to grow. The first chemist of the USDA, Charles M. Wetherill, went rogue by exploring the idea of food adulteration. Wetherill wanted to determine if he could adulterate wine by adding sugar to grape juice to increase the alcohol content. His detour resulted in the creation of an entirely new department, the Bureau of Chemistry, which would later become the FDA.[2,4] Over time, the organization continued to grow. Today, the FDA employs over 15,000 people and is funded by the taxpayer to the tune of $4.4 billion a year.[5] However, in the 1860s, the FDA (the Bureau of Chemistry at the time) was a sleepy organization. It didn't have a lot of money or authority.

Meanwhile, our food supply was undergoing rapid changes. In the late 1800s and early 1900s, the Industrial Revolution ushered in a new age where families left their farms in exchange for life in the city. Consequently, our diets changed dramatically. As we moved off farms, we transitioned from eating farm-fresh foods to a reliance on processed and canned foods. Instead of cooking our food ourselves, we began relying more on other people and companies who would prepare food for us in distant cities. We became separated from our food supply, which put us in a difficult position.

There were no labeling laws. Companies were not legally required to tell you what was in that can of corn beef hash you were eating. Therefore, consumers had to blindly trust the manufacturing companies if they wanted to eat their products, which was a scary proposition because manufacturers had begun adding more preservatives to our foods to prevent them from rotting on the shelves. Some of the preservatives included: benzoic acid (aka borax), salicylic acid, formaldehyde, sodium benzoate, and copper salts. At the time, benzoic acid was used to cure and preserve meat because it could reduce the smell of bad meat;

copper sulfate made faded vegetables appear green again; and sodium benzoate prevented tomatoes from rotting.[4,6]

These chemicals were not tested for safety, so nobody knew if they were dangerous for us to eat. Nobody knew what levels, if any, were safe and what level would be considered poisonous to humans. And, since the manufacturers decided which chemicals to put in our food and how much, they held all the cards. In addition, there were no legal consequences or penalties if a company sold chemical-laden foods. Thus, the opportunity to adulterate our food supply existed and consumers were aware of it. But, public concern wasn't strong enough to support a federal food law or a federal agency that would oversee our entire food supply.

That didn't stop people from trying to centralize our food supply. In 1880, the chief chemist at the Bureau of Chemistry (FDA) was Peter Collier. After he conducted an investigation on food adulteration, Collier recommended that Congress pass a national food and drug law. At that time, there were inferior foods of low quality labeled under high quality names. Essentially, people figured out how to make fakes and then labeled them as the real deal. For example, adding brown coloring and a dead bee into a jar of glucose created honey. Adding brown coloring and a pinch of flavoring to glucose could make maple syrup.[6] In addition, colors that were poisonous were added to candies.[7] In light of the numerous instances of food adulteration, Collier determined that regulations were needed at a national level. Consequently, a bill was drafted, but it was defeated in Congress. During the next 25 years, over 100 food and drug bills were proposed with the intent of creating a centralized regulation of our food supply. All of the bills were defeated. All efforts failed until Dr. Harvey W. Wiley entered the scene.

Dr. Wiley was a Republican who wanted the federal government to regulate businesses, at least food manufacturers. He was on a mission to eradicate adulteration from our food supply. His crusade began while working as a professor at Purdue University. In Dr. Wiley's first published paper on food adulteration, he argued that honey was contaminated when glucose was added to it.[4] Later, in 1883, he was appointed as the head of the Bureau of Chemistry (FDA). Dr. Wiley longed for the opportunity to test food additives for safety. In 1902, he got his chance. Congress gave $5,000 to the Bureau of Chemistry (FDA) to study the effect of chemical preservatives and colors on digestion and health.[8] Dr. Wiley used the money to expanded the agency's food adulteration studies by creating a "poison squad", where healthy young men would become guinea pigs.[8] According to renowned historian Dr. Larry Schweikart:

> "The men were monitored as they ingested food laced with ever-increasing doses of additives, which, of course, produced side effects. In what would typify government's haste to 'fix something' before completely contemplating all ramifications, Harvey [Dr. Wiley] sent the volunteers off to their meals with no consent forms, no animal studies, no lab tests, and no institutional medical oversight. They ate large doses of borax, salicylic acid, formaldehyde, sodium benzoate, and copper salts, swallowed in gelatin capsules halfway through their meals, making 'several men so sick they couldn't function'."[4]

Dr. Wiley continued to test chemicals on young men for five years.[4] According to the FDA, "He stopped each unconventional experiment after many of his volunteers became sick."[7] Consequently, Dr. Wiley concluded that every chemical he tested in his study should be banned. To his disappointment, only formaldehyde was.[4]

After conducting many experiments, Dr. Wiley made three major recommendations:

1. Chemical preservatives should only be used when necessary.
2. Food producers should be responsible for ensuring the safety of their products.
3. Consumers have the right to know what they are eating.

Dr. Wiley's recommendations would eventually become the backbone of our national food laws and regulations, but America still wasn't ready for a centralized beauracracy.[7] He did, however, successfully alert the public to the seriousness of the food adulteration problem in America. And, his studies did increase public support for a national food law. According to one of the Wiley's supporters:

> "The picture of that little 'Poison Squad' in Washington swallowing its daily doses of borax caught first the fancy of the press and then that of the public. In a few months a single sensational venture did what twenty-three preceding years of laborious toil had failed to accomplish."[9]

But, it still wasn't enough. Dr. Wiley would need help convincing Americans to hand over the regulation and oversight of their food to the federal government. He would receive it from an unsuspecting source: a book. One book struck fear straight through the hearts of Americans. It would leave them sickened, outraged, and demanding federal oversight of their own food supply.

## Sucker Punch

Upton Sinclair wrote a book called *The Jungle,* which led directly to an attack on meat. It resulted in the "first full-fledged government offensive against a food group."[4] The outcome of this anti-meat campaign would change our entire system of food oversight and regulation. It gave birth to our modern governmental structure that oversees our food supply, the FDA. The outrage stemming from Sinclair's book was the final piece of the puzzle that Dr. Wiley needed to achieve his goal of a centrally regulated food supply. And, it was all an accident.

Sinclair wasn't trying to get a food law passed or help forge the path for the formation of the FDA. He was trying to tug at the hearts of Americans to garner support for socialism. Sinclair famously stated, "I aimed for the public's heart and by accident hit it in the stomach."[10]

Sinclair was a self-professed socialist. In 1903, he joined the socialist party and later ran for governor of California on the socialist ticket. He envisioned a peaceful revolution where capitalism would be overthrown and the government would take ownership of big businesses. He thought that if he could touch the hearts of Americans, they would eagerly and voluntarily vote for fundamental change. Sinclair got his chance when the leading socialist magazine in the country, *Appeal to Reason,* hired him in 1904 to write an exposé on the meat-packers union strike.[11,12]

Journalism was changing at that time. It began to play an important role in exposing wrongdoing, partly because publishers realized that sales soared when they featured stories about political corruption and corporate misconduct.[12] Consequently, *Appeal to Reason* paid Upton Sinclair $500 to write a piece about the meat-packers strike, including the unfair labor conditions of the meat-packing workers.[11,12] But, Sinclair had a different idea in mind.

Sinclair wanted to write a book that would have as much influence as *Uncle Tom's Cabin,* an 1852 anti-slavery novel by Harriet Beecher Stowe that sparked public outcry and support for the war to free the slaves.[10]

Sinclair wanted to do the same for workers in America, which he viewed as slaves to the capitalist system.[10] Thus, at the age of 26, he dedicated nine months of his life to his assignment. When he was finished, Sinclair had written a political manifesto that promoted socialism over capitalism. Based on a fictional plot, *The Jungle* was his socialist rally cry.

*The Jungle* follows the hardships of a Lithuanian man named Jurgis who immigrated to Chicago with his family. He gets a job in the meatpacking district of Packingtown as a "shoveler of guts."[13] He ends up losing his finger on the job. With no workers' compensation and no responsibility claimed by the employer, Jurgis' life falls apart. He loses his wife, son, house, and job. The destruction of his family unit is blamed on the corrupt and oppressive meatpacking industry i.e. capitalism. Then, one day, Jurgis hears a speech about socialism. He attends socialist political rallies that inspire him to support their cause. These speeches are Sinclairs' own dreams of American "workers voting for socialist candidates to take over the government and end the evils of capitalist greed."[11] The book closes with his rally cry: "Organize! Organize! Organize!" so that "Chicago will be ours! *Chicago will be ours!* CHICAGO WILL BE OURS!"[13]

Much to Sinclair's disappointment, Americans did not rally behind the plight of the meatpacking workers nor did they flock to the socialist party. Instead, Americans fixated on his deplorable depictions of the meat itself. Almost as an afterthought, Sinclair wrote a few pages about diseased, rotten, and contaminated meat products that were treated with chemicals to mask their decaying stench and flavor, and then deceptively mislabeled and sold to Americans as food. He also alleged that some meatpackers would process diseased animals into meat when no meat inspectors were around.[11] Even though Sinclair only dedicated a handful of pages to the adulteration of the meat supply, Americans were so sickened and outraged that it completely overshadowed his goal of shining light on the unfair working conditions. As Sinclair himself realized, with grave disappointment, his novel "hit [Americans] in the stomach" and not in the heart as he had originally intended.[10]

Nonetheless, *The Jungle* was an instant success. It sold one million copies in its first year of publication, became an international best seller, and was published in 17 languages.[11,14] It even made it to the big screen as a silent film in 1914. The movie poster was provocative, picturing a man falling into a vat of steaming lard. *The Jungle* was so influential during its' day that it is still required reading in many history and literature classes. When I was required to read that book in high school, I was so grossed out that I refused to eat hamburgers for months! I never imagined that our food supply could have been so adulterated and so dangerous. It was a shocking revelation for me. I remember reading about piles of meat in dark rooms where:

> "...thousands of rats would race about on it. It was too dark in these storage places to see well, but a man could run his hand over these piles of meat and sweep off handfuls of the dried dung of rats."[13]

The rats were allegedly ground up in the meat. There were stories about workers urinating next to meat and workers with tuberculosis coughing and spitting blood on the floor where meat was kept. Sinclair even alleged that workers at the meat packing facility would sometimes fall in the steaming vats of lard and be ground up and sold to Americans as food.

> ". . and when they were fished out, there was never enough of them left to be worth exhibiting,--sometimes they would be overlooked for days, till all but the bones of them had gone out to the world as Durham's Pure Leaf Lard!"[13]

These types of descriptions of the adulterated food supply ensured the success of *The Jungle,* as well as the fallout. Soon after its release, the White House was bombarded with phone calls and letters from Americans demanding reform. "Women's organizations from around the country and the American Medical Association (AMA) threatened everything including a march on the offices of the congressional leaders if no action was taken [that] year," according to the FDA.[6] The public outcry was so large that it forced Congress and the President of the United States to act quickly.

## Congress Enters The Jungle

When *The Jungle* was published in January of 1906, Dr. Wiley's Pure Food and Drugs bill was stalled in Congress. Even though Dr. Wiley was still lobbying for his bill and even though President Theodore Roosevelt encouraged Congress to pass it, there was opposition from conservatives and industry, namely food processing and drug companies. *The Jungle* changed all of that.[12]

Roughly one month after *The Jungle* was published, the Senate overwhelmingly approved the Pure Food and Drugs Act by a vote of 63 to 4. But, the bill did not include any provision for meat inspection. So, Senator Albert Beveridge, a progressive Republican from Indiana, proposed a second bill that would require federal inspections of meat that crossed state lines. In addition, the Department of Agriculture would regulate the packinghouses and a federal inspector would be present on-site at all hours of operation.[12,15] Senator Beveridge declared his bill to be, "the most pronounced extension of federal power in every direction ever enacted." The Senate approved his bill.[12]

Both bills passed the House after Senator Beveridge agreed to give up the provision that required a date to be stamped on all canned meat. Interestingly, product dating of meat is still not required by the USDA.[16] In addition, if a company chooses to date their product, there is still no agreed-upon standard.[16] Regardless, after getting through Congress, the bills landed on the desk of President Roosevelt who signed them both into law on the same day. June 30, 1906 was a historic day in America when both the Meat Inspection Act and the Pure Food and Drugs Act became law.[12]

How did both the Senate and the House pass these two bills so quickly? Surely the meatpacking companies had lobbyists on Capitol Hill ready to defeat any bill that could hurt or impede the meat industry. Couldn't they have defeated or at least slowed down the passage of the bill? It turns out that the large meatpacking companies strongly *supported* the Meat Inspection Act.[17] They wanted new regulations on the books. Why would a business want more government "red tape"? Why would the large meatpacking companies want Big Brother looking over their shoulder all day, every day?

It's a way to crush the smaller competitors. Do you recall my experience working for a large supplement company? They wanted more regulations because it's more difficult for a smaller company to keep up with the cost of business when more government regulations are imposed. Likewise, the large meat-packing companies supported more government regulations to help stomp out their smaller competitors.[18]

The large meatpacking companies had another incentive as well. Not only would a new regulatory law crush smaller competitors, it would increase profits. Meat sales were cut in half following the release of *The Jungle,* so the meat industry was looking to increase consumer confidence in meat.[19] A new law that placed a government watchdog inside industry and put the government seal of approval on meat would allay public fears that were incited by *The Jungle*. But, here's the real kicker. The big meatpacking companies managed to get *us* to pay for their inspections! Taxpayers picked up the entire $3 million bill. It was $3 million in 1906. Today, the price tag is $1.2 billion.[20] And yes, we still pay the bill.

In the end, Americans got the federal regulations they were screaming for, in addition to the $3 million tab. The large meatpacking companies got free inspections that would increase consumer confidence in meat, and new regulations that would help stomp out their smaller competitors. Dr. Wiley finally got his Pure Food and Drugs Act passed after battling on Capitol Hill for over a quarter century. President Roosevelt gained more control over corporations, which made him very happy. He declared these two laws, in addition to a bill that regulated railroad rates, to be "a noteworthy advance in the policy of securing Federal supervision and control over corporations."[12] And, Upton Sinclair helped pass two of the most influential pieces of legislation in our history. He must have been thrilled, right?

Wrong.

Sinclair opposed the Meat Inspection Act! He knew it was designed to favor the big meat packers. In the end, Sinclair "had been a fool and a sucker who ended up being used by the very industry he hated,"[18] according to the Foundation for Economic Education.

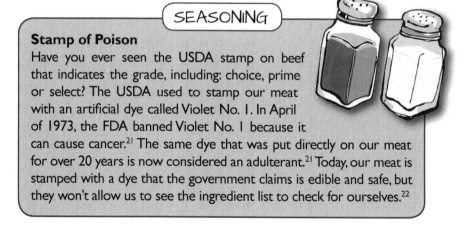

## SEASONING

**Stamp of Poison**
Have you ever seen the USDA stamp on beef that indicates the grade, including: choice, prime or select? The USDA used to stamp our meat with an artificial dye called Violet No. 1. In April of 1973, the FDA banned Violet No. 1 because it can cause cancer.[21] The same dye that was put directly on our meat for over 20 years is now considered an adulterant.[21] Today, our meat is stamped with a dye that the government claims is edible and safe, but they won't allow us to see the ingredient list to check for ourselves.[22]

## 1906: The Year Of The Veil

The Meat Inspection Act and the Pure Food and Drugs Act ushered in a new, unprecedented era of government regulation of our food. These two bills are considered to be the **birth of the FDA**, and are sometimes given credit for the birth of our modern day federal government.

The Meat Inspection Act prohibited the sale of mislabeled or adulterated livestock and required sanitary conditions during slaughter.[23] It also allowed the government to inspect meat that was sold across state lines.[7] It was truly a power grab by the federal government.

The Pure Food and Drugs Act prohibited "the manufacture, sale, or transportation of adulterated or misbranded or poisonous or deleterious foods, drugs or medicines, and liquors."[24] It was "a centerpiece of progressive reforms in the early 20th century."[24] It ended up being "the most consequential regulatory statute in the history of the United States."[14] The 1906 Pure Food and Drugs Act was so significant that, in 1998, the U.S. Post Office commemorated its passage on a stamp.[2]

The passage of these **two food laws permanently changed who controlled our food supply.** In 1906, the regulatory reigns were taken from the states and local governments and handed over to the federal government. When *The Jungle* was published, there were already some state and federal meat inspections in place. For instance, the USDA inspected pork exports beginning in the early 1890s. However, the Meat Inspection Act took government oversight to a whole new level. It placed federal inspectors in all packinghouses any time the meat was destined to be sold between state lines or to foreign countries.[25] In other words, the federal government would be on-site all the time. In addition, the Pure Food and Drugs Act gave the federal government authority to regulate the manufacture and sale of food. It was "the most daunting intrusion by federal authorities into interstate commerce."[14] On that historic day of June 30th, the authority over our food supply was placed in the firm grip of the federal government, namely the FDA and the USDA.

Amidst our fears of canned goods laced with poison and meat contaminated with rat poop and human fingers, the federal government swooped in to save the day. By swiftly enacting new laws and regulations that were touted to protect the consumer, and by placing a government watchdog in meat packing plants at virtually all hours, consumer confidence in the food supply would resume. In addition, our relationship with our food supply would permanently change. According to the

FDA, the Pure Food and Drugs Act provided "basic elements of protection that consumers had never known before that time."[2] There's the rub! There's the **birth of the veil of unearned trust**. Once the federal government became the watchdog over our food supply, Americans breathed a sigh of relief as they began to wash their hands of the responsibility of ensuring the safety of the foods they ate.

The media reinforced the perception of the federal government as the heroic do-gooder ushering in a new era of safe food. "Congratulations" was plastered on editorial pages across the county and the *New York Times* declared, "The purity and honesty of the food and medicines of the people are guaranteed."[6] 'Guaranteed,' now that's a strong word. I can see the veil of unearned trust falling over the eyes of Americans.

The new government food regulations ushered in a false sense of security across America. Government regulation "leads [the consumer] to assume that they are being protected by the government, reducing the incentive to do their own checking," according to the Foundation for Economic Education.[17] For instance, because federal inspectors were placed in every meatpacking plant, people felt safe. However, this change would lead to an unintended consequence.

The government inspectors tested the meat by using a "poke-and-sniff" method. Inspectors would literally poke a rod into the meat and smell it. If it smelled clean, the inspector would poke the same rod into the next slab of meat. This method was used to test the meat throughout the entire plant. An obvious flaw with this method is that you can't typically smell pathogens until they have grown large enough in number to produce a detectable odor.[15] "USDA inspectors undoubtedly transmitted harmful bacteria from one contaminated piece of meat to other uncontaminated pieces in untold quantities and, consequently, were directly responsible for sickening untold numbers of Americans by their actions," according to the Northeastern University Law Journal.[26] Did the government regulations protect or harm Americans in this situation?

The "poke-and-sniff" method remained the "centerpiece of the USDA's meat inspection program until the late 1990s."[26] How do you feel about the veil of trust now? "Poke-and-sniff" is no longer the "centerpiece," but it is still used by the USDA when inspecting our meat. It's combined with other "safety" testing, including observing plant employees and company records, along with occasional microbial testing.[27]

Think about it: When was the last time you looked into the safety of your meat? Do you know where your meat is raised or processed, or how it is inspected? That's the veil. It began to fall over the eyes of Americans in 1906, and it continues today.

SEASONING

## Arsenic in your chicken?
Arsenic used to be commonly added to chicken and turkey feed in America.[28] It helps them grow faster and it gives the meat a healthy pink coloring. But, arsenic ended up in the meat that we eat. That's bad because arsenic is a known carcinogen, meaning it can cause cancer.[29] The European Union banned feed additives containing arsenic in 1999, but America didn't.[29] However, there is some good news. The FDA withdrew approval of 98 arsenic-based animal drugs in 2013 after being sued by the Center for Food Safety and eight other groups.[28] Later, in 2015, the last arsenic-based animal drug was removed from the market.[28]

## Built On Lies?

It's easy to blame the American people for ushering in the modern era of centralized food oversight and regulation. But, let's remember that they were acting out of fear. In addition to hearing Dr. Wiley's warnings about poisonous food additives, Upton Sinclair sent fear through the hearts of Americans with his claims about their adulterated meat supply. If I learned that I was eating ground up humans and rats, I would probably scream for regulation and oversight as well, at least initially. Regardless, the people certainly got what they wished for.

There's only one small problem. *The Jungle* might have been based on lies! Some people argue that Upton Sinclair never visited a meatpacking house. According to the Foundation for Economic Education,

> "Sinclair relied heavily both on his own imagination and on the hearsay of others. He did not even pretend that he had actually witnessed the horrendous conditions he ascribed to Chicago packinghouses, nor to have verified them, nor to have derived them from any official records."[18]

The words of renowned historian Dr. Schweikart echo this sentiment:

"...Sinclair never bothered to go to a Chicago packing-house to see conditions for himself, choosing instead to rely on the assertions of others."[4]

Even President Roosevelt didn't trust Sinclair. Roosevelt wrote a letter to journalist William Allen stating, "I have an utter contempt for him. He is hysterical, unbalanced, and untruthful."[4,18] Roosevelt declared Sinclair's book to be full of lies:

"Three-fourths of the things he said were absolute falsehoods. For some of the remainder there was only a basis of truth."[4]

Roosevelt wanted to find out for himself what was going on in the meatpacking industry. So, he sent an investigative team to Chicago. The Department of Agriculture's Bureau of Animal Husbandry conducted the first investigation. Their report refuted Sinclair's most outrageous accusations, calling them "willful and deliberate misrepresentations of fact," "atrocious exaggeration," and "not at all characteristic."[18] Consequently, President Roosevelt wrote a letter to Frank Doubleday, the owner of the company who published Sinclair's book, blasting him for publishing "such an obnoxious book." The publisher backed the claims made by Sinclair in *The Jungle*. So, Roosevelt launched a second investigation.[12] This time he appointed labor commissioner Charles P. Neill and social worker James Bronson Reynolds to check out the conditions. Neither had any experience in the meatpacking business.[18] After visiting Chicago, Neill and Reynolds confirmed Sinclair's claims, which meant there were now two conflicting reports, both conducted by government employees. Who would Roosevelt believe?

Roosevelt ended up using the report from Neill and Reynolds so he could strong-arm the Senate into passing the Meat Inspection Act. He threatened to release the findings of the report if they didn't act. Consequently, the Senate promptly passed the bill. Later, Neill and Reynolds would testify that they had an agenda. They admitted that they wanted to find fault with the meatpacking industry so a new inspection law could be passed.[18] It might be a coincidence, but the timing worked out well for the economy since meat sales had dropped by half in the United States within just weeks of the publication of *The Jungle*.[6]

I don't know if Sinclair was sensationalizing or if the government was covering their behinds, but the evidence is stacked against Sinclair. For example, we know that before Sinclair's book was published in 1906, local, state and federal governments had been inspecting meat for a decade and had never reported a single complaint.[4] In addition, Congressman E. D. Crumpacker of Indiana testified in June of 1906 that none of the government officials employed to inspect meat "ever registered any complaint…with respect to the manner of the slaughtering or preparation of meat or food products."[18] Besides, roughly 2 million visitors toured the Chicago stockyards and packinghouses every year.[30] Surely, someone would have alerted the authorities or the public if the conditions were as bad as described in Sinclair's book.

In addition, Sinclair wrote a second book that he touted as truth, but later admitted was based on a lie. Roughly 20 years after *The Jungle* was released, Sinclair wrote a book titled *Boston*, which he also hoped would fuel the socialist movement. In a letter to John Beardsley, Sinclair admitted that *Boston* was based on a lie.[31] Having done it once before, is it really unbelievable to think Sinclair might have bent the truth in *The Jungle*?

Regardless, in the court of public opinion, *The Jungle* provided the push that was needed for Americans to accept federal oversight of our food supply. It's crazy to think that such a fundamental change in the structure of America occurred largely because of a book that was most likely based on lies.

SEASONING

**Bath Time!**
The chicken in your local grocery store has probably taken a bath in chlorine. To kill pathogens, the USDA allows our chicken to be washed with chlorine.[32] Nobody knows how much chlorine residue remains on the chicken and how much ends up on your dinner plate. This practice is banned in the European Union.[29] Europe won't even allow American chicken to be sold to their citizens if it's been treated with chlorine.[29]

HANDS OFF MY FOOD!

Together, Dr. Wiley, Upton Sinclair, and President Roosevelt helped forge the way for the FDA to take a prominent and leading role in the centralization of our food regulation and oversight. Two laws ushered in an unprecedented expansion of federal power.[10] With the USDA serving as its' sidekick, the FDA became the watchdog over our food, triggering the lowering of the veil of unearned trust over the eyes of Americans.

## The Whole Thing Is Unconstitutional!

"The Food and Drug Administration is unconstitutional."[33]

—Michael Farris,
Constitutional attorney and
Founder of Patrick Henry College in Virginia

Based on the original intent of the Commerce Clause (Article I, Section 8 of the Constitution of the United States), the federal government has authority to regulate international imports and the shipment of goods across state lines.[33] The Commerce Clause limits the authority of the federal government by reserving the regulatory power over the food supply to the states and the people. In fact, prior to the 20th Century, that's how the food supply in America was regulated: The federal government was mostly limited to regulating imported food, while state governments regulated domestically produced and distributed foods.[5] That relationship changed with the birth of the FDA.

The FDA is an unconstitutional over-reach of authority by the federal government. It exists through a distorted interpretation of the Commerce Clause.[33] Since the FDA is unconstitutional, all rules and regulations imposed on the American people by the FDA that do not involve imports or shipping foods across state lines are unconstitutional, if we follow the Constitution's original meaning.[33]

Therefore, "The 1906 Meat Inspection Act is unconstitutional," according to Constitutional attorney Michael Farris.[33] The Meat Inspection Act is an over-reach of authority by the federal government. It became a law based on a misinterpretation of the Commerce Clause. The Commerce Clause gives the federal government authority to regulate the shipment of goods across state lines. That means the government can regulate planes, trains and ships. But, the Commerce Clause does not give government authority to regulate what occurs inside manufacturing facilities, such as farms. Consequently, placing federal meat inspectors inside of meat processing plants is unconstitutional.[33]

SEASONING

## Food Fight

The first national anti-food campaign in America targeted alcohol. In 1919, our country had just emerged from World War I and temperance groups "played on [Americans] fears of moral decay."[34] It was our fear that led to the ratification of the 18th Amendment to the U.S. Constitution.[35] For the first time in our history, a food was banned on the national level. Think about that for a moment: Our government passed a Constitutional amendment that made it illegal for us to consume a particular food. Why would we ever give government that authority? Prohibition eroded our individual liberty, but it also eroded states' rights by taking regulatory authority from the states and local governments and handing it directly to the federal government. Did you know the 18th Amendment is the only Constitutional amendment that restricts freedom? All of the other amendments either guarantee our freedoms or define them.[36]

## Take Home Message

Both the Food and Drugs Act and the Meat Inspection Act of 1906 became law largely because of a poison squad and a sensationalized book. In a state of fear, the people turned to the federal government for help. Consequently, 1906 was the year that *permanently* changed the American food supply. In that revolutionary year, the regulatory reigns over our food were taken from the states and local governments and handed to a centralized authority, namely the FDA. It was also the year that permanently changed our relationship with our food supply. Once the federal government became our watchdog, Americans breathed a sigh of relief as they began to wash their hands of their responsibility to ensure the safety of their own food.

1906 was the year the veil of unearned trust began to fall over the eyes of Americans. It's been handed down with each generation, like a family heirloom. Over time, as the federal government has grown, so has our veil. Today, it remains firmly fixed over our eyes. It's thicker than it has ever been and the consequences it brings are more detrimental to our Nation, our health, and our freedom than ever before.

## Moving Forward

Now that we know how the veil came to be, let's take one more step and ask ourselves a difficult question:

### What are the consequences of abdicating our responsibility over our food supply?

I contend that our food supply is more adulterated and dangerous today than it has ever been in the history of our nation. We've trusted the government, industry, and "experts" with our food for over 100 years, and look at where it has gotten us:

- Our government largely decides what we eat for dinner and how much it costs.
- We eat untested and unregulated chemicals in our food every day. The FDA knows and they say it's not their problem.
- We are un-consenting guinea pigs because the FDA doesn't think we have the right to know when companies put *experimental* products on the market.
- Industry is pushing genetically modified crops and genetically modified animals onto our dinner plates without conducting toxicity or long-term safety studies. Not only did the FDA help industry get these "foods" on the market, they don't think we have the right to know we are eating foods that have been *fundamentally* changed at the gene level.
- The government nudges us, on a daily basis, to eat foods that are making us sick. We're losing our health and our freedom by allowing the government to change our perception of food.

In the next 5 chapters, I will expand upon these truths in more detail. Along the way, let's ask ourselves:

- Is the FDA "protecting and promoting your health?"
- Is industry putting your long-term health in front of their short-term gains?
- Are "experts" seeking scientific truths or are they pursuing an agenda?
- Have industry, government, and "experts" earned your trust?

**Or, is it time to reclaim your role as watchdog over your food supply?**

SECTION 2:


# WHAT GOVERNMENT AND INDUSTRY
# ARE DOING TO OUR FOOD

# CHAPTER 5:

# SUBSIDIES

### *Government Chooses Your Dinner For You*

"Lawmakers would be hard-pressed to enact a set of policies that are more destructive to farmers, taxpayers, and consumers than the current farm policies."

—Brian M. Riedl, Heritage Foundation

Have you ever wondered why fruits and vegetables are more expensive than chips, soda, and cookies? Last week, I paid $9.98 for a bag of organic grapes, yet a box of Oreos® containing 36 cookies costs less than $3.00. Why is healthy food typically more expensive than processed junk food?

The answer is quite simple: The Farm Bill.

We should all care about the Farm Bill because it is arguably the most influential food law in American history.[1] This one bill, which was crafted by politicians and lobbyists, largely determines what's on your dinner plate *and* how much it costs. It's the reason Oreos® are so much cheaper than grapes.

Until recently, I avoided learning anything about the Farm Bill. It's long, it's filled with complicated Washington D.C. lingo, and I didn't think it made a difference in my life. After all, I'm not a farmer so why should I care about the Farm Bill? I was wrong, completely wrong.

## It's All Connected

"The Farm Bill connects the food on our plates, the farmers and ranchers who produce that food, and the natural resources-our soil, air and water-that mak[e] growing food possible. In the simplest terms, the Farm Bill has a tremendous impact on farming livelihoods, how food is grown, and what kinds of food are grown. This in turn affects the environment, local economies, and public health."[2]

-National Sustainable Agriculture Coalition

## The Corn Illusion

The federal government largely decides what's on your dinner plate by picking winners and losers. Through the modern Farm Bill, our government pays farmers who grow certain crops. For instance, in the United States, roughly 300 million acres of land are planted with food. Half are dedicated to corn and soy, while 50 million are for wheat, 11 million are used to grow our fruits and vegetables, and the remainder is used for other field crops such as rice, cotton, and barley.[3] Why is two-thirds of the farmland in America used to grow corn, soy, and wheat?

Farmers are paid to grow these crops. Over 90% of farm subsidies are given to farmers that grow just five crops, including: corn, soybeans, wheat, rice, and cotton.[4]

As crop variety has decreased, so have our food choices. Here's how it works: With so many farmers growing the five subsidized crops, particularly corn and soy, Americans end up with more of these foods than they can eat. That surplus drops the price of these five commodities, leaving farmers with a bunch of cheap crops on their hands. What happens with the surplus of cheap crops?

They are converted into cheap, synthetic byproducts and then added to our processed foods. These cheap man-made chemicals replace the relatively more expensive natural ingredients, the type you might find in your kitchen.

Let's look at corn as an example, since it is the most heavily subsidized crop in the U.S.[5] You may think you don't consume much corn.

After all, when was the last time you ate corn on the cob or popcorn? Unfortunately, thanks to the Farm Bill, it's not that simple any more.

If you think you're safe from the long-reaching tentacles of corn, think again. The American diet is riddled with corn. Walk into your local grocery store and you will be greeted with the obvious culprits: corn on the cob in the produce section, and popcorn and corn chips in the snack aisle. But, continue walking down the snack aisle and you will find corn in your favorite packaged crackers and cookies. Yep, corn is even in our cookies! It's used for flavoring and to increase the shelf life of products. It can even be in the vanilla extract that is added to our chocolate chip cookies, and the baking powder that makes our cakes light and fluffy.

Hop on over to the cereal section and you will find yourself staring at rows of corn. Since corn can be present in artificial or natural flavoring, your cereal is almost certain to contain corn. Walk further down the grocery store aisle and say hello to the corn in your favorite salad dressing. Yep, even salad isn't safe from the long-reaching tentacles of corn. It's a common thickening agent in dressings, soups, puddings, and sauces, including mayonnaise and pasta sauce. It can even be in your spaghetti noodles! If you buy bread to eat with your pasta dinner, get ready for another dose of corn. Bread can contain corn in the form of malt flavoring and mono- and diglycerides. And, if your bread is fortified or enriched, it probably contains corn because corn derivatives are used to make vitamins and minerals.

Head over to the frozen food section and you'll arrive at a dinner party with a special VIP section for corn. Corn oil is often used to fry your chicken nuggets, corn dogs, and egg rolls. Corn is used as a meat filler and thickener in frozen meals. It's even in your frozen seafood! Some wild fish are dipped in a solution containing corn syrup or corn derivatives before they are frozen.

Visit the meat department and you're in for a real treat; it's one big pile of corn. Chickens, pigs, cows, and even some fish, are fed large amounts of corn and corn by-products.[6,7] That corn becomes part of the drumstick, steak, or fillet that ends up on your dinner plate. But, the corn feast doesn't stop there! Corn derivatives such as vinegar and lactic acid are often used to clean the meat before it's packaged for our consumption. Even chicken eggs contain corn. All dairy products, including milk, cheese and yogurt, contain corn unless the cow was fed its' natural diet of grass.

Grab a soda to wash down your meal and you are drinking liquid corn in the form of high fructose corn syrup. Most people already know that, but did you know that fruit juice often contains corn? And, what about the orange juice you buy specifically because it contains added vitamin C? That vitamin C is probably made from corn. And, let's not forget the beer! Alcohol can be made using fermented sugar that was made from cornstarch. Munch on some pretzels with that beer and you'll get a pinch of corn in the form of salt. That's right, even iodized salt can contain corn.

In the mood for dessert? Walk over to the bakery and you'll find corn in the powdered sugar that coats your doughnuts. It can also be in the icing that tops your cakes and cupcakes. If you think you can escape corn by opting for ice cream, think again. Corn is used to thicken ice cream! Corn is even in sugar-free candy in the form of xylitol. It can also be in honey! Some bees are fed high fructose corn syrup, which means corn ends up in the honey. You can't even escape corn if you buy a fresh apple. Apples are typically coated with wax to make them look better. Guess what the wax is made from?

Yep, corn!

As you can see, when you walk down the aisles of your local grocery store, corn literally surrounds you on all sides. Your store may appear to have a huge variety of foods to pick from, but it's an illusion. What you are really choosing between is different variations of re-packaged corn byproducts. Why? Why does our food contain so many processed corn ingredients and byproducts?

Because they are cheap thanks to government subsidies.

Through the Farm Bill, government incentivizes U.S. farmers to grow corn, and it works. America is the world's largest corn producer, growing 90 million acres of corn each year.[8] Consumers can only eat so much corn, so what happens to the extra?

Most of the surplus corn is processed into feed for our livestock. Some is exported to other countries. Some is converted to ethanol and burned as fuel.[9] Yep, we burn food as fuel. The rest of the surplus corn is processed into chemicals that we likely eat on a daily basis. Some of these chemicals include: high fructose corn syrup, xanthan gum, maltodextrin, cellulose, and lactic acid. There are hundreds of synthetic chemicals, made from corn, that are added to our food. Some of these synthetic chemicals have replaced natural alternatives. Let's take a closer look at high fructose corn syrup (HFCS), since it's currently abundant in our food supply.

The USDA credits the development of HFCS to the government farm program. According to the USDA, "Government programs have been instrumental in the development of the HFCS."[8] The story of HFCS began when a Japanese scientist named Yoshiyuki Takasaki created a form of HFCS in a laboratory in the 1960s. In 1966, a corn processing company was granted an exclusive license to manufacture HFCS from *Streptomyces* bacteria.[10] The company began selling their HFCS product for use in our foods the next year; however, the use of HFCS didn't accelerate until after the FDA determined it to be "generally recognized as safe" or GRAS in 1976 (We will discuss the GRAS loophole in a subsequent chapter).[11] It was around this time when food manufacturers realized they could cut costs by replacing ingredients that you would typically find in your kitchen, like pure cane sugar, with ingredients that were subsidized, like HFCS derived from corn.[12] Consequently, pure cane sugar was kicked to the curb as HFCS became the new king of sugar. And Americans gobbled it up!

In the 1970s, Americans ate 5.5 pounds of HFCS per person per year. By the year 2000, our appetite grew to 63.8 pounds per person per year![13] Today, over 8% of our daily calories come from HFCS while less than 1% comes from vegetables.[14,15] You may not even realize how much HFCS you eat because it can appear in a whole slew of processed foods including: soup, canned fruit, yogurt, crackers, cookies, cereals, salad dressing, pizza sauce, bread, soda, and even peanut butter.

This system of swapping natural ingredients for cheaper subsidized ingredients can be credited to Secretary of Agriculture Earl Butz. It was his 1970s farm policy that "sharpened its focus on creating cheap raw materials. It turned farmers from tenders of the land into managers of agribusiness."[16] Butz oversaw a food revolution that was so successful in creating cheap raw materials that our annual consumption of corn *more than doubled* between the 1970s and 2000, from 11 pounds per person to 28.4 pounds.[13] **Americans now eat corn on a *daily* basis in the form of processed corn byproducts.**

It's no surprise that cheaper synthetic chemicals, like HFCS, have replaced natural sources of sugar in our foods. It's a cost-savings decision made by companies. What did surprise me was learning why these alternatives are cheaper. The lower cost is not just because the government subsidizes corn. It's also because the U.S. government keeps the price of cane and beet sugar artificially high. We have the Farm Bill to thank for that as well.

The 1981 Farm Bill came with a gift for taxpayers: a new government program called the U.S. sugar program. According to the USDA, "The U.S. sugar program uses price supports, domestic marketing allotments, and tariff-rate quotas…to influence the amount of sugar available to the U.S. market. The program supports U.S. sugar prices above comparable levels in the world market."[17]

In other words, the federal sugar program keeps the price of natural sugar artificially high to guarantee U.S. sugar producers a profit. The government accomplishes this goal by guaranteeing a certain price for U.S. sugar crops and by taxing (through tariffs) sugar imports. For instance, in 2006, sugar producers were guaranteed 22.9 cents per pound for beet sugar and 18 cents per pound for cane sugar, even though the world price for cane sugar was only 10 cents per pound. That means Americans paid roughly "double the world price for sugar."[18]

The government also keeps domestic sugar prices artificially high by burning "excess" imported sugar. The 2008 Farm Bill gave us the sugar-to-ethanol program. Under this program, the government sells sugar to ethanol producers who turn it into ethanol for use as fuel in cars. One person, the Secretary of Agriculture, controls how much sugar will be burned. The purpose of the program is to help American sugar growers maintain control of over 85% of the U.S. sugar market by preventing "downward pressure on inflated domestic sugar prices."[19] In other words, consumers lose again because our government keeps sugar prices artificially inflated by mandating the "surplus" be burned as fuel.

If the "sugar protection" was removed, the cost of sugar-containing products, like baked goods and soft drinks, would be even lower than current prices, according to *Reason* magazine.[18] In addition, if natural sugars were not artificially inflated in price, some manufacturers might return to using natural sources of sugar instead of the laboratory chemicals that are currently added to our favorite cookies and crackers. After all, the replacement of pure cane sugar with synthetic HFCS occurred largely because of the environment our government created. By incentivizing the production of a handful of cheap crops and by artificially inflating prices, the government created a surplus of cheap ingredients. This incentivized industry to replace more expensive natural ingredients, like pure cane sugar, with cheaper subsidized ingredients, like HFCS. And, it's not just corn that has taken over our processed foods. Let's meet corn's partner in crime: soy.

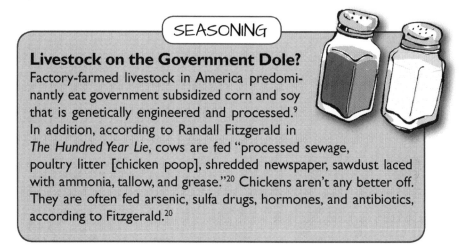

SEASONING

**Livestock on the Government Dole?**
Factory-farmed livestock in America predominantly eat government subsidized corn and soy that is genetically engineered and processed.[9] In addition, according to Randall Fitzgerald in *The Hundred Year Lie*, cows are fed "processed sewage, poultry litter [chicken poop], shredded newspaper, sawdust laced with ammonia, tallow, and grease."[20] Chickens aren't any better off. They are often fed arsenic, sulfa drugs, hormones, and antibiotics, according to Fitzgerald.[20]

## "Corn Chips" With A Dollop of Soy[21]

Not only do we eat a lot of processed corn, Americans eat a lot of processed soy. Government-subsidized soy takes a close second to corn, with over 77 million acres planted every year.[22] Since we can only eat and export so much soy, the surplus is processed into soy byproducts such as: vegetable oil, soy protein, textured vegetable protein, and lecithin. Just as in the case of corn, these byproducts are readily added to our processed foods and animal feeds. In fact, soybeans account for roughly 10% of the total calories in our diets.[23] So, while the supermarket shelves appear to contain a vast selection of foods ranging from Asian to Mexican to Greek, they are really just variations of the same foodstuffs: processed corn and soy. By incentivizing farmers to grow just a handful of crops, the government has effectively decreased the diversity of our diet without us even knowing.

To make matters worse, the majority of that corn you eat is genetically engineered. That means the corn you eat today is not the same corn you grew up eating. Now it has genes from a bacteria inserted into it. And, it's not just corn. Three of the five most subsidized crops, including soy and cotton, are largely genetically engineered and a fourth is in the works. In total, over 90% of all corn, soy, and cotton planted in the United States is genetically engineered.[24] These three government-subsidized crops take up roughly 169 million acres of farmland.[25] That means roughly half of all the land used to grow our food is planted with genetically engineered crops.[25] We're eating those crops, as processed byproducts, without knowing it. Even the USDA admits that Americans don't know they are eating genetically engineered foods:

> "More than 15 years later, adoption of these varieties by U.S. farmers is widespread and U.S. consumers eat many products derived from GE [Genetically Engineered] crops…largely unaware that these products were derived from GE crops."[25]

We may be "largely unaware," but that's because the FDA thinks we don't have the right to know (We will discuss this deception in chapter 8).

Both genetically engineered and processed corn and soy byproducts are added to our processed foods in abundance. Since the average American consumes 75% of their calories from processed foods and beverages, that means the government has selected a dinner for you that consists of genetically engineered, processed corn with a side of genetically engineered, processed soy.[15] But wait, it gets worse.

By picking winners and losers, the government has not only chosen your dinner, it has chosen what chemicals *your body* is made up of. You literally are what you eat. The foods you eat are broken down in your gastrointestinal tract, absorbed into your blood stream, and incorporated into your tissues. Therefore, the foods you eat literally become your body, including your brain, heart, muscles, lungs, and all of your other organs and tissues. What's disturbing is that Americans eat so much corn, due largely to government subsidies, that **we are turning into corn** and scientists can "prove" it.

Scientists can measure how much corn we eat by testing our hair for a specific type of carbon contained in corn. According to a researcher at the University of California at Berkeley, the hair of a typical American contains 69% of its carbon from corn.[23] That means we are predominantly made up of genetically modified, processed corn! In fact, Americans are made up of more corn than Mexicans, who traditionally eat a corn-based diet.[21] As Michael Pollan, author of *Omnivore's Dilemma*, famously wrote, we are "corn chips with legs."[21] And don't forget about all of the processed soy we eat. In essence, **we are genetically** engineered "corn chips" with a dollop of genetically engineered soy on top.[21] But, is that really a bad thing?

According to a recent study conducted by the Center for Disease Control (CDC), the answer is yes. In 2016, the CDC published a study in *JAMA Internal Medicine*, one of the most reputable scientific journals. According to the study, "People who ate more of these subsidized foods were more likely to be obese, register high levels of bad cholesterol, and have high blood sugar and inflammation."[5,26] How much subsidized food did the 10,308 study participants eat? 56% of their daily calories came from subsidized food commodities.[26] That number may seem high, but it's pretty typical for Americans. Remember, we consume roughly 75% of our calories from processed foods and now our own government (the CDC) is telling us that this food is making us sick.[27] How do you feel about those farm subsidies now?

We could spend this entire book debating the question of whether or not it's bad for Americans to eat too much processed corn and soy, but the answer doesn't matter for the purpose of this book. My goal is not to convince you that eating lots of processed and genetically modified corn and soy is bad for your health. That's an individual decision that you can make for yourself. The point I'm making is this:

- The Farm Bill drives down the price of synthetic food ingredients while the government artificially inflates the price of natural alternatives.
- This incentivizes industry to use the cheaper synthetic ingredients in our cakes, cookies, crackers, pizzas and other processed foods.
- If you eat like a typical American, who consumes 75% of their calories from processed foods and beverages, the government has largely picked your dinner for you.

It's like we are all standing in the frozen food section deciding between Mexican and Asian food for dinner. What we don't realize is that the decision has already been made for us. We are really choosing between genetically engineered processed corn and soy or genetically engineered processed corn and soy. Both frozen dinners are just variations of the same foodstuffs: synthetic, genetically engineered, subsidized byproducts.

What does this mean in terms of individual liberty?

## A Link Between Food and Disease

Let's take a closer look at how a subsidized crop could affect your health. What you eat has a profound effect on your overall health and wellbeing because the food you eat literally becomes your body. In my opinion, each person is an individual so we cannot know, with 100% certainty, which foods are "good" for you and which foods are "bad" for you. Thus, "experts" draw generalized conclusions about individual foods. For example, omega-6 fats are generally pro-inflammatory while omega-3 fats are anti-inflammatory.[28] Consequently, if you eat too many omega-6 fats and not enough omega-3 fats, your body could become inflamed.[28] That's bad because nearly every disease is associated with inflammation, including heart disease, cancer, diabetes, and autoimmune conditions.[28,29] Guess which foods are rich in omega-6 fats? Corn and soy.

## Loss Of Authority Over Our Choices And Our Bodies

When you eat like a typical American, you have lost some authority over your own food choices. Each time you eat subsidized food, you are consenting to be a genetically engineered "corn chip with legs" with a dollop of genetically engineered soy on top.[21] You are consenting to allow the government to decide which chemicals you are made of. In doing so, you are allowing the government to determine, in part, your long-term health and wellbeing. It's a scary predicament we find ourselves in, especially when you realize that the CDC has declared subsidized foods to contribute to disease.[26] But, don't worry. If you choose to eat lots of subsidized byproducts and you get sick, the government has a plan: You can rest easy knowing that government funded healthcare is available in the form of Medicare, Medicaid and the Affordable Care Act in the event that the government subsidized food makes you sick.

Welcome to the new "circle of life" in modern day America, where taxpayers foot the bill to make cheap processed food. Then, taxpayers foot the bill again to heal the people who get sick from the subsidized food. All of us have already bought into this system on some level. It's a system that uses our own tax dollars against us by making healthy food expensive and potentially unhealthy food cheap. And, it's built on hypocrisy.

## The Hypocrisy Of Subsidized Food

What's most interesting to me regarding our Farm Bill is the hypocrisy. Our government-issued dietary guidelines recommend we eat less junk food, including processed food. The former Surgeon General, Dr. Richard Carmona, linked processed food to our current obesity epidemic.[30] According to Dr. Carmona, "Obesity is the terror within" and "unless we do something about it, the magnitude of the dilemma will dwarf 9-11 or any other terrorist attempt."[31] Do you see the hypocrisy?

The government tells us that processed foods lead to disease and we should eat less of them, but they subsidize the very same food that they claim is making us sick. They create and enforce agricultural policies that are in direct opposition to their own dietary recommendations. For instance, our government guidelines suggest you fill half of your plate with fruits and vegetables. However, historically, less than 1% of the Farm Bill budget has been set aside to support these crops.[32] Instead, the money supports the commodity crops that are used to make cheap junk food. According to Politico:

> "If you were to create a MyPlate meal [the new Food Pyramid] that matched where the government historically aimed its subsidies, you'd get a lecture from your doctor. More than three-quarters of your plate would be taken up by a massive corn fritter (80 percent of benefits go to corn, grains and soy oil). You'd have a Dixie cup of milk (dairy gets 3 percent), a hamburger the size of a half dollar (livestock: 2 percent), two peas (fruits and vegetables: 0.45 percent) and an after-dinner cigarette (tobacco: 2 percent). Oh, and a really big linen napkin (cotton: 13 percent) to dab your lips."[32]

### And, the government uses our tax dollars to fund their hypocrisy!

In addition, while propping up a system that creates cheap junk food, our government drives up the price of fruits and vegetables.[33] For instance, incentivizing farmers to grow a handful of commodity crops discourages them from growing fruits and vegetables because the guaranteed money is in subsidized crops. To put it another way: Would you plant the crop that guarantees you money or would you plant the crop that could bankrupt you if it fails? Less fruits and vegetables are grown in the United States partly because the guaranteed source of income is dangled over the farms that produce commodity crops.[33]

That's largely why fruits and vegetables are relatively more expensive than junk food. In fact, the indexed price of fruits and vegetables has increased 40% since 1980. In contrast, the price of soda dropped 30% during the same time period.[34] According to Congressman Tim Ryan:

> "…as a member of the United States Congress I have…watched many public setbacks as our government continues policies and strategies that make eating bad food or fake food the most convenient option."[35]

### Our tax dollars help make junk food cheaper and healthy food more expensive.

Have you been in the produce section lately? Vegetables and fruits are expensive compared with processed cereals, cake mixes, and some bread. In fact, an obesity researcher from the University of Washington wanted to figure out why lower-income individuals are more likely to be overweight than wealthier individuals. He learned that $1 could buy 1,200 calories in cookies or potato chips, but that same dollar could only buy 250 calories in carrots. In addition, that $1 could buy 875 calories in soda, but only 170 calories in orange juice.[36]

It's the government who largely determines the cost of your dinner, and it's primarily because of the Farm Bill. It's actually a simple concept: The junk food is cheaper than healthy food because it is made with ingredients that the government pays farmers to grow. In *The New York Times Magazine*, Michael Pollan argued that the reason a Twinkie® is less expensive than a pack of carrots, in spite of the fact that the Twinkie® contains nearly 40 ingredients and undergoes a high-tech manufacturing process, is because "the Twinkie is basically a clever arrangement of carbohydrates and fats teased out of corn, soybeans and wheat–three of the five commodity crops that the farm bill supports..."[36] It's crazy to think that a Twinkie® is cheaper than a small pack of carrots. After all, the Twinkie® has 40 times the ingredients and those ingredients have to be shipped to a processing plant, processed into chemicals, combined with other ingredients to be made into a Twinkie®, packaged, and then shipped to market. That entire process is cheaper then pulling a carrot out of the ground. That's the Farm Bill in action. Scratch that, that's the government in action!

SEASONING

### Arsenic in Rice!
The government subsidizes rice, which means rice gets added to many of our processed foods, including baby foods. This is concerning because rice reportedly contains inorganic arsenic, which can be toxic. According to the FDA, "Consumption of inorganic arsenic has been associated with cancer, skin lesions, cardiovascular disease and diabetes in humans."[37] How did arsenic get in our rice?

Some arsenic is naturally present in soil. However, inorganic arsenic was used as a pesticide in America until it was banned in the 1980s. And, some arsenic residues still remain in the soil today.[38] Since rice is grown in water-flooded conditions, and arsenic is water-soluble, the rice sucks up the arsenic. Consequently, it's showing up in our crackers, cereals, and even baby food. The FDA found "significant levels of inorganic arsenic in rice and rice cereals, including rice cereals for infants."[37] That's a problem since chronic exposure to arsenic can result in cognitive impairment and early disease in children.[39]

The FDA has proposed a limit on the amount of inorganic arsenic allowed in infant rice cereal; however, it's merely a suggested limit. Companies are under no obligation to adhere to the FDA recommendation.[40] Across the top of the FDA document that contains the suggested arsenic limit, it states "Contains Nonbinding Recommendations."[37]

## All Roads Lead To "We The People"

The federal government might have orchestrated the new American "circle of life," but it ends with us. Allow me to explain.

The government pays farmers who agree to grow certain crops. What do you think farmers are going to do in this situation?

They are probably going to grow the government crops so they can get paid. It's hard to blame them. Farming is a risky business. Weather, insects, and disease can wipe out your entire crop, taking your income with it. If someone offered you guaranteed money and all you had to do was plant the crops they wanted, would you take the deal?

Many farmers took the deal. In exchange for financial security, farmers gave up crop variety. Traditionally, farmers managed the inherent risk of farming, in part, by planting a variety of crops. For instance, if your broccoli crops failed, you could still rely on your strawberries, tomatoes, and cauliflower to bring in your income. That changed with the Farm Bill. By incentivizing farmers to grow just a handful of crops, that's exactly what we got: rows and rows of cheap surplus corn and soybeans.

Meanwhile, the government incentivized industry to add the cheap surplus ingredients to our processed foods by driving down their cost while artificially inflating the cost of natural alternatives. In turn, industry accepted the risk of possible long-term health consequences for their customers in exchange for their short-term gains. Remember our Doritos® example?

It's easy to blame farmers or industry for making decisions based on cost, but let's first consider our own food choices. What role do we play in this equation?

While the government largely picks your dinner for you, including the cost, **you give your consent.** Roughly 75% of the American diet is made up of processed foods instead of whole foods, like fruits and vegetables.[15] In addition, over one-third of our calories come from junk food, including items like cookies and candy.[41] We make those choices. We choose to eat junk food instead of vegetables. We choose the convenience of processed foods.

I believe cost is a big reason for the shift in our food choices away from whole foods and towards subsidized foods. Processed foods are simply cheaper, so your money goes further when buying those subsidized foods. Just like industry, **government has incentivized you** to choose the cheaper junk foods. Think about it: Have you ever said that you wanted to eat better, but you didn't because "healthy" food is too expensive? Our decisions as consumers largely boil down to cost-savings.

In that sense, we are no different than industry when we decide to risk the possible long-term health consequences in exchange for the short-term gains. We'll take the cheaper foods now with the hope that we don't suffer from food related health issues later. In doing so, we buy into the government "circle of life." While the government incentivizes us to choose the cheaper foods, they don't force us to eat them. We make those decisions as individuals. Each time we eat subsidized food, we accept the associated health risks, but we also give our consent to the government-created "circle of life." With each bite, we speak with our dollars.

In fact, if your goal is to be cost-effective in your food choices and you don't care about the possible long-term health consequences or your dollars supporting government subsidies, your best bet is to eat a lot of government subsidized foods. Your money simply goes further when buying those foods. For that matter, the typical American who eats at least 75% of their calories from processed foods should be applauded for gaming the system! They are receiving the maximum short-term financial return on their purchase. In contrast, people like me who don't eat government subsidized processed foods are the losers in this system. I am paying, via my tax dollars, to make the food cheaper for everyone else that does eat subsidized food.

In addition to giving our consent, we play another role in the new "circle of life." **We help determine which crops are planted and how much are planted.** For instance, our decision to eat 75% of our calories from processed foods lowers the demand for fruits and vegetables, which contributes to raising their price. Very little acreage in the U.S. is allotted to growing fruits and vegetables compared to subsidized crops, which results in relatively less supply. With less supply comes a higher price. This is an example of how our food choices affect the market. Yes, the government decision to subsidize a handful of crops has increased acreage of those crops while decreasing acreage of fruits and vegetables; however, **we bought into the system.** We made the individual decision to change our eating habits from whole foods to highly processed foods. In doing so, we consented to the government subsidies program by buying the products that system created. As long as we continue to choose subsidized food at the expense of whole food, the "circle of life" will continue.

## Lunch Time!

Children are the real losers when it comes to the Farm Bill. They are stuck eating the highly-processed foods that the government has encouraged our farmers to overproduce. According to Michael Pollan, "The farm bill essentially treats our children as a human Disposall for all the unhealthful calories that the farm bill has encouraged American farmers to overproduce."[36] After the surplus crops are processed into food-like substances, including junk food and other processed foods, they are used in the nutrition programs at schools. These processed foods become our children's school lunches. And, it's not just wheat, corn, and soy that are subsidized in school lunches.

Have you ever wondered why our government pushes milk on us, particularly on our children?

The government subsidizes milk. To be accurate, taxpayers subsidize the milk used in school lunches. We spent $4 billion in the last 10 years on milk.[33] That's a lot of milk money! Just as we saw with subsidized crops, the government had to figure out what to do with the surplus milk that came with government subsidies. So, the USDA decided to dump it on our children.

That solution worked for a while, but milk production in America increased every year since 2010, reaching over 208 billion pounds in 2015.[42] So much milk was produced in 2015 that processing plants couldn't keep up with the supply. Consequently, some dairies dumped the surplus milk into pits used for livestock manure.[43] The surplus milk was literally dumped on the ground. Our tax dollars paid for that spilt milk!

To add insult to injury, as taxpayers, **we are charged twice** for the foods subsidized in our children's lunches. We pay farmers through the federal subsidies included in the Farm Bill. After these crops are processed into food-like substances, we pay another tax when the subsidized junk foods are used in the nutrition programs at schools.[16] In other words, first we subsidize the crops, like wheat and corn, and then we buy them back to be used in our children's lunches. It's a double tax. But, the food taxes don't end there.

**We pay a third tax** on the inflated food prices that are created by the government farm policies. Let's take milk, for example. Not only do we pay farmers to produce milk and then buy the milk for school lunches, we buy it at an artificially inflated price. Our government intentionally keeps the price of dairy, including milk, artificially elevated. Like sugar, dairy enjoys price supports and trade barriers in the U.S. Therefore, it's estimated that the average price of U.S. nonfat dry milk was 23% more than world prices, cheese was 37% higher, and butter was roughly twice the cost between 2000 and 2002.[18]

The bottom line is that the Farm Bill keeps food prices high, except for the handful of government-selected commodities.[18] In 2004, the Organization for Economic Cooperation and Development estimated that the U.S. farm policies pushed food prices higher by $16.2 billion. Guess who paid the bill?

We did!

According to *Reason magazine*, that price tag was "an annual 'food tax' per household of $146."[18] What would you do with an extra $146 in your pocket?

That raises another question: The Farm Bill costs taxpayers between $15 and $35 billion each year.[19] Where is all that money going?

## Millionaires And Dead People

In theory, the Farm Bill is a program that helps keep the agricultural sector and our food supply stable and affordable. It works through price supports as well as loans and insurance payments to help farmers defend against adverse weather, pests, and price fluctuations. However, the reality of the program is not so pretty. Let's take a look at how much this monstrous program costs taxpayers and who is benefitting.

Total farm support ranges from $15 billion to $35 billion each year.[19] Between 1995 and 2012, tax payers coughed up $292 billion to subsidize the farm program.[35] Where did all of that tax money go?

According to *The Week*, the Farm Bill "keeps food prices high, costing consumer billions, while funneling most of its aid to giant agribusinesses and wealthy farmers. While we are paying more for our artificially inflated food, we are also paying Big Ag to stay big. Roughly 75 percent of total subsidies go to the biggest 10 percent of farming companies."[44]

As corn and wheat subsidies have increased over the decades, the Farm Bill has disproportionately benefitted Big Ag while small farmers have been left out to dry. The distribution of government funds is so skewed that *The Week* declared the Farm Bill to be "a welfare program for millionaires and giant agribusinesses." For instance, taxpayers spend roughly "$25 billion annually to subsidize a small, elite group of farmers through policies that do nothing to help the farm economy," according to the Heritage Foundation.[45]

This was not the original intent of the Farm Bill. According to the *New York Times*, farm subsidies were originally an anti-poverty program but have evolved into government handouts for the top 1% of farms:

"FARM subsidies were much more sensible when they began eight decades ago, in 1933, at a time when more than 40 percent of Americans lived in rural areas. Farm incomes had fallen by about a half in the first three years of the Great Depression. In that context, the subsidies were an anti-poverty program. Now, though, the farm subsidies serve a quite different purpose. From 1995 to 2012, 1 percent of farms received about $1.5 million each, which is more than a quarter of all subsidies... Some three-quarters of the subsidies went to just 10 percent of farms. These farms received an average of more than $30,000 a year."[46]

**Our tax dollars helped squeeze out the family farms and give rise to Big Ag.** "Subsidizing well-heeled agribusiness interests has ensured the continued exodus of independent family farmers from the land... In the United States, family farmers have been sold out to corporate agribusiness with ever-increasing numbers of farm bankruptcies and foreclosures," according to *Foreign Policy in Focus*.[47] There you have it, the birth of Big Ag: The farming industrialized complex that the political left loves to hate was an unintended consequence of the Farm Bill, which is a bill that was enacted by the Democrats.[33]

In addition to Big Ag, **our tax dollars are given to millionaires who claim to be farmers**. According to the IRS and the GAO, between 2003 and 2009, millionaires received over $316 million in farm program payments.[48] You may recall hearing about "fake farmers" in the news, including Bruce Springsteen, Jon Bon Jovi, Ted Turner, and U.S. Representative and former Eagles tackle Jon Runyan.[44] Americans on both sides of the political aisle were outraged as we learned that Bon Jovi only paid $104 in taxes on 7.1 acres of land because he hired someone to raise bees.[49] In addition, Mark F. Rockefeller was paid $342,634 to *not* farm on his land from 2001 to 2011.[44] Yep, you read that right. We gave our tax dollars to an heir of the Rockefeller fortune so that he would not farm.

Let's be very clear on this point: These millionaires are not doing anything illegal. It might be morally wrong, but the problem is the farm subsidies. These subsidies are so misguided and so massive that our tax dollars are now supporting millionaires who decide to become "fake farmers," as well as millionaires who want to idle their land. In fact, according to the GAO, the farm program is so mismanaged that $1.1 billion was paid to dead farmers over a six-year period. Specifically, 172,801 deceased farmers received tax dollars through the Farm Bill; 40% of these recipients had been dead for 3 or more years.[50]

Our tax dollars are also given to homeowners that live on land that used to be farmland. For instance, a housing development was built on 75-acres of former Texas farmland. Because the land was previously used to grow rice, the government continues to send checks to the homeowners. "Some of them collect hundreds of thousands of dollars without planting a seed,"[51] according to the *Washington Post*. A few have asked the government to stop sending the checks, but they keep coming. Sadly, this waste of our tax dollars is not isolated to Texas. It's estimated that since 2000, $1.3 billion in farm subsidies has been handed to people across the United States who don't farm.[51,52] According to *The Washington Post*, "The cash comes with so few restrictions that subdivision developers who buy farmland advertise that homeowners can collect farm subsidies on their new back yards."[51] That means we are literally paying for some homeowners to grow grass in their backyards! The Farm Bill has become so mismanaged, misguided, and filled with loopholes that even *The Washington Post*, a left-leaning news organization, said it should be vetoed![53] So, why do we still have the Farm Bill?

SEASONING

**Farmers Paid Not to Farm**
The original Farm Bill of 1933 restricted the amount of food farmers could grow by paying them not to farm. To participate in the program, farmers were required to keep a portion of their farmland on reserve where no crops would be grown.[4]
Who wouldn't want to participate? The farm program took the risk out of farming by providing farmers with a guaranteed income for not working. It was a short-term win for farmers. It was also a win for our government because it allowed them to control the supply of crops. The original crop choices included: wheat, rice, corn, cotton, and tobacco. The government actually paid farmers *not* to grow these crops. Hogs and milk were also subsidized.[54]

One government official, the Secretary of Agriculture, decided how much farmland each farmer was required to idle.[4] The Secretary was also given authority, under the Farm Bill, to set food prices for each crop (in the form of a conversion factor), to determine how much tax should be imposed on processors to pay for the Farm Bill, and to decide how much tax money would be given to participating farmers. That's an enormous amount of authority entrusted to one individual.

When the Food Bill was passed in 1933, Henry A. Wallace was handed that authority. What would he do with so much control over our agricultural sector? He would grow the government. Wallace created the Agricultural Adjustment Administration, which was put in charge of the monstrous farm program. But, he didn't stop there. Under his watch, Wallace grew the USDA to an unprecedented size. He turned a small government agency into "one of the largest arms of the government, with more than 146,000 employees and a budget of more than $1 billion. (USDA Farm Bill budgets now average nearly $90 billion.)"[4] Wallace was rewarded for his efforts when he was selected to serve as vice president under President Roosevelt during his third term in office in 1941.

## Never Let An "Emergency" Go To Waste

The Farm Bill was supposed to be a "temporary solution to deal with an emergency," according to Secretary of Agriculture Henry Wallace.[55] American food production greatly increased during World War I. Farmers took out loans to keep up with demand. However, when global markets rebounded after the war ended, the demand for American food exports dropped. Consequently, food prices fell, leaving farmers with a surplus of crops along with a pile of debt. Then, the Great Depression hit and the rough times quickly grew worse for farmers.[56]

At the time, roughly 25% of the population lived on farms and their income suddenly plummeted.[45] President Franklin Delano Roosevelt vowed to "wage a war against the emergency."[1] Within his first few days in office, Roosevelt won passage of the first Farm Bill, officially known as the Agricultural Adjustment Act of 1933. That one bill *permanently* changed the federal government's relationship with our farmers and our entire agricultural sector.[1] For the first time, Congress declared it was the job of the government to balance supply and demand of our farm crops.[57] **The farm crop free market was officially dead.**

The Farm Bill was supposed to end when the "emergency" ended. As written in the Farm Bill, the act would be terminated "whenever the President finds and proclaims that the national economic emergency in relation to agriculture has been ended…"[54] Today, roughly 1% of people living in America are farmers. And, "the average farm household earns $81,420 annually (29 percent above the national average); [and] has a net worth of $838,875 (more than eight times the national average)," according to the Heritage Foundation.[52] The emergency is over, yet the Farm Bill remains.

## Unconstitutional

According to Michael Farris, Constitutional attorney and founder of Patrick Henry College, "The Farm Bill is unconstitutional."[58] Specifically, the federal government does not have authority to regulate agricultural production. The Supreme Court agreed.

In 1936, in the case of *United States v. Butler*, the Supreme Court ruled that it was unconstitutional for the federal government to set target prices.[4] The authority to regulate agriculture, according to the Supreme Court, remains with the states.[59] Specifically, the Supreme Court opinion declared:

> "The regulation is not in fact voluntary. The farmer, of course, may refuse to comply, but the price of such refusal is the loss of benefits. The amount offered is intended to be sufficient to exert pressure on him to agree to the proposed regulation. The power to confer or withhold unlimited benefits is the power to coerce or destroy…It is clear that the Department of Agriculture has properly described the plan as one to keep a non-cooperating minority in line. This is coercion by economic pressure. The asserted power of choice is illusory."[60]

The ruling temporarily halted the farm assistance program, but it didn't stop it. After tweaking the language, Congress passed a new Farm Bill that remains the foundation of our current agricultural policy.

## Government Kills Pregnant Pigs While Americans Starve

Instead of allowing for a free market, our government created a centralized food policy centered on their ability to control the supply of our food. The goal of the first Farm Bill was to restore "the purchasing power of farmers."[54] To accomplish that goal, the government needed to increase the value of crops. They reasoned that if supply decreased then crop prices would increase, effectively putting money in the pockets of farmers. How would the government decrease the supply of existing crops?

They destroyed the surplus crops. One of the first objectives of the program when it was created in 1933 was to plow up 10 million acres of cotton.[56] Within the first year of the program, 25% of cotton crops were successfully destroyed.[61] The government destroyed livestock as well. As part of an emergency slaughter program, 9 million pounds of pork were destroyed.[56] Even sows about to give birth to baby pigs were killed. One million sows were slaughtered by our government, an event the press dubbed "the killing of little pigs."[61]

Americans were outraged when they learned that their own government was destroying food while bread lines, soup kitchens, and homelessness had become a common sight. Americans were starving while our government was throwing away food. In response to the public outrage, a new government program was established, the USDA Surplus Disposal Program. It's purpose was to give the surplus food to families in need.

## Lobbyists Control Washington

It's no surprise that industry helps push the Farm Bill through Congress each time it's up for renewal. They have a lot to gain from this one bill, and so they spend a lot of money on lobbyists to ensure they receive their share of the pie. It's hard to blame them. Under the current Farm Bill, the government has become a huge money piñata. Whoever shows up to the party with the biggest bat gets the most candy. Big Ag and Big Food bring telephone poles.

Between 2009 and 2013, Big Food spent $185 million on federal lobbying. Big Ag spent $111.5 million lobbying for the 2013 Senate Farm Bill. In total, the agricultural sector spent nearly $150 million on lobbying in 2013 alone.[35] What do they lobby for?

According to Congressman Tim Ryan in *The Real Food Revolution,* a hefty sum of money was spent to convince the American people that subsidized foods, like high fructose corn syrup, are good for us to eat:

> "One example of the strength of the corporate lobbying dollar is the Corn Refiners Association (CRA), a trade association that is made up of six giant corporations, including Cargill and Archer Daniels Midland. In recent years, the CRA has been spending tons of money to promote a positive image for high-fructose corn syrup. Between 2000 and 2013, the CRA spent approximately $5.2 million in federal lobbying. It was also revealed that the CRA spent more than $30 million on a private PR campaign, including $10 million to fund a four-year research project by a cardiologist that disputed the contention that there are any negative health consequences from corn-based sweeteners!"[35]

In addition, lobby money is used to influence government rules and regulations:

> "Cargill spent $1.4 million in 2013 lobbying on crop production and processing issues, with specific issues listed as 'poultry processing, partially hydrogenated vegetable oil rulemaking, food labeling and claims, food additive regulations, pathogen regulation, antibiotics.'"[35]

**Lobbyists don't just sway politicians, they help write the Farm Bill.**[52] According to the Center for Responsive Politics, a non-profit watchdog on federal lobbying dollars, 325 organizations and individuals who worked on the 2013 Senate Farm Bill were registered as lobbyists.[62]

## When Two Worlds Collide

It should not be surprising that rural legislators support the Farm Bill, however I was surprised to learn that some urban legislators do too. Why would urban politicians support a bill that gives money to farmers? Their constituents live in cites. That just didn't make sense. Then

I learned that **the Farm Bill includes other government programs, including food stamps and school lunches**. In fact, *most* of the funding for the Farm Bill is allotted to food assistance programs. According to a Congressional Research Service report, "food aid topped [the] 2008 farm bill spending," gobbling up a whopping 67% of the budget. In contrast, only 15% of the budget was spent on commodities.[63] In 2014, food aid topped the Farm Bill budget again, eating up nearly 80% of the tax-payer funds.[64]

Once urban and rural legislators joined forces, the Farm Bill became practically untouchable. According to Chris Edwards of the Cato Institute, this unlikely partnership translates into an ever-growing USDA budget with the taxpayers on the hook:

> "While farmers are a smaller share of the population today than in the 1930s, the farm lobby is perhaps as strong as ever. One reason is that farm-state legislators have co-opted the support of urban legislators, who seek increased subsidies in agriculture bills for programs such as food stamps. Legislators interested in rural environmental subsidies have also been co-opted as supporters of farm bills. Thus many legislators have an interest in increasing the USDA's budget, but there are few opposing them on behalf of the taxpayer."[4]

Now that the Farm Bill has been "co-opted," legislators have little or no incentive to reform it or, better yet, stop renewing it. No Congressman is going to oppose the Farm Bill when it brings so much money to their constituents, unless they don't want to get re-elected. Besides, some members of Congress who vote on the Farm Bill have received farm subsidies, including: Senator Charles Grassley (R-IA), Senator Gordon Smith (R-OR), and Representative John Salazar (D-CO).[52]

The Farm Bill also plays a major role in the Presidential election. Agricultural policies are a primary issue for voters in rural counties and states. Consequently, as the candidates compete for the 270 electoral votes needed to win the Presidency, agriculture takes center stage.[65] This is particularly true of Iowa, which is the first state to pick a Presidential nominee. Simply put: If you want to win Iowa, you may not want to oppose the Farm Bill.

Some people say that the Farm Bill is here to stay. It certainly may seem that way: Big Food and Big Ag are incentivized to lobby the

HANDS OFF MY FOOD!

government because it has become a big money piñata. Legislators are incentivized to push through the Farm Bill because it brings money to their constituents, which helps them get re-elected. And taxpayers are footing the bill to the tune of roughly $30 billion each year. But, that's a victimized view of the situation. Let's not forget about the powerful role we play, both as voters and consumers.

## What You Can Do

If you'd like to take action against the Farm Bill, here are some ideas:

- **As consumers**, every time you eat you have a choice: You can continue to buy the genetically engineered and processed subsidized food, which supports the Farm Bill. Or, you can buy more whole foods like fruits, vegetables, beans, nuts, and seeds. If we stop buying the foods that support the Farm Bill, or even try to buy less of them, we can make a difference. We can help change the market by shifting demand, which shifts supply. Every bite counts. Here are some ideas to get you started:
  - Consider eating one meal each day that does not contain any of the five most subsidized crops (corn, soy, wheat, rice, and cotton). For instance, instead of processed spaghetti noodles made from wheat, try spaghetti squash. Or, leave the bun off your burger and add a vegetable to your plate.
  - If you're not ready to change a full meal then try one snack. For example, instead of corn chips, grab an apple or a banana. Instead of cheese on crackers, try nut butter on celery.
  - You can also choose drinks that don't contain high fructose corn syrup. Instead of a soda made with HFCS, choose one made with pure cane sugar. Alternatively, choose water or real fruit juice with no added sugar.
  - If your child attends school, you can opt-out of the school lunch program. Instead, provide a packed lunch filled with whole foods.
  - If you attend church and they provide processed snacks for the children, ask them to provide fruit instead. If cost is an issue, ask parents to donate money to the cause. An organic apple costs less than $1 and it stays fresh for several days in a refrigerator.

- **As voters**, we can use our voice to end, or at least restrict, the Farm Bill:
  - Stop electing Congressmen and Presidents who support the Farm Bill. As long as they keep getting re-elected, they will keep voting for this monstrous bill that you and I pay for. If you want to know how your Congressman voted on the Farm Bill, you can visit this website: www.govtrack.us.
  - Since the Farm Bill distorts the agricultural market, it will be challenging to use the free market to get rid of it. However, there is another option. We can restrict the power and jurisdiction of the federal government. Based on Article V of the United States Constitution, "We the People" can call for a convention of states. Through a convention, we can restore the checks and balances on federal power thereby eliminating programs, including the Farm Bill, which are an unconstitutional over-reach of the federal government. This is a controversial solution. Each of us must decide for ourselves if this is the correct path for our Nation. For more information, please visit www.conventionofstates.com.

## Take Home Message

In 1933, the first Farm Bill was sold to the American people as a "temporary solution to deal with an emergency."[55] It's still alive and kicking today. For over 80 years, our tax dollars have funded a centralized food program that allows the government to pick winners and losers. By distorting the market, and artificially inflating food prices, the government has largely chosen what's on our dinner plates and how much it costs. Since you are what you eat, Americans are literally genetically engineered and processed "corn chips" with a dollop of genetically engineered and processed soy on top.[21]

Using the Farm Bill, the government incentivizes farmers to grow government-selected crops, they incentivize businesses to add the processed surplus to our foods, and they incentivize consumers to eat processed foods by driving down the cost. The real losers are the people: The government uses our tax dollars to make subsidized processed food cheap, and it's making us sick![26]

It's a frustrating system, but it's important to remember that the real power remains with the people. **Only the people can change our**

**food supply.** We can vote out the Congressmen who support the Farm Bill, but we can also make a difference on a daily basis. If we learn to consciously speak with our dollars, we can slowly move the agricultural market. Change can happen and it starts one bite at a time.

> "The large corporations at the heart of the current food system, supported by our government, dictate what's available to eat at what price. If it's not working for you, you need to fight back."[35]
> —Congressman Tim Ryan

## Moving Forward

Now that you know who chooses your dinner for you, in addition to the price tag, let's turn our attention to the synthetic chemicals lurking in our food. These chemicals are made in a laboratory. They are not safety tested or regulated by the government.[66] Yet, they are so abundant in our food supply that most Americans eat them every day. Here's the real kicker: It's legal! The FDA knows about it and they say it's not their problem. In the next chapter, we'll discuss the *one* loophole that is literally poisoning our food supply.

CHAPTER 6:

# GRAS

## *The Loophole That Poisons Our Food*

"Rules governing the chemicals that go into a tennis racket are more stringent than [rules for] the chemicals that go into our food…At least when you put a new chemical on the market, you have to notify the EPA. But there's no requirement that you notify the FDA when you make a new food additive."[1]

—Thomas Neltner,
Director of the Food Additives Project,
Pew Charitable Trusts

Have you read the ingredient list of your favorite food? It can be like reading from a chemistry book: propylparaben in Sara Lee® cinnamon rolls, butylated hydroxyanisole (BHA) in Contadina® pizza sauce, and propyl gallate in Pop Secret® popcorn.[2] I recently flipped over a box of Pillsbury® bread mix and saw ingredients that I could hardly pronounce, including butylated hydroxytoluene (BHT) and propylene glycol. It's crazy when you take a step back and realize that a chemist is sitting in a laboratory right now, creating the next chemical† that will end up on our dinner plates. What's even crazier is that many of us will

---

† The term "chemical" is used to describe products sold by additive manufacturers. Sometimes these chemicals are referred to as ingredients, additives, or substances, which are all technically chemicals, or are a mixture of chemicals.

blindly eat it! Even though we know these chemicals are synthetic and we can't even pronounce their names, we still eat them. Why?

We assume that someone is making sure these chemicals are safe. Even if we don't trust the food manufacturers, we trust the government oversight of our food supply. Think about it: When was the last time you walked into a grocery store and questioned if the food was safe? Would you question if your box of Cheerios® or bag of Oreos® was safe to eat? How about a bread mix sold by Pillsbury®? Many of us don't give the safety of these foods a second thought. Instead, we fall back on the belief that the chemicals in our food are safe to eat because the government is regulating them. After all, if the government allows these chemicals in our foods they *must* be safe, right?

Since most Americans eat foods containing synthetic chemicals, I contend that most of us believe they are safe.

But, is our belief system built on truth?

There are roughly 10,000 chemical additives in our food supply.[3] Should we blindly trust them? In other words, does the government really test those chemicals for safety or are we part of an unplanned nationwide experiment conducted by chemical companies?

## Shattered Beliefs

The typical American eats approximately 75% of their calories from processed foods, which means **most of us eat synthetic chemicals every day**.[4] They are used to make processed foods taste good and look appealing. When whole foods are processed, they frequently lose their taste and color. So, companies add those qualities back to the food using *synthetic* chemicals, called food additives. Additives are also used to preserve foods so they can sit on grocery store shelves longer. Additionally, additives are used to package, store, and transport food.[3] They make our lives easier and more convenient, but they come at a price.

BHT in the Pillsbury® bread mix, for example, helps preserve the mix so it can sit on the grocery store shelf. But, it is also used in embalming fluid and jet fuel.[5] And, it's associated with DNA damage, inflammation, and tumor promotion.[6-9] Propyl gallate in Pop Secret® Popcorn helps prevent fat from going rancid. But, studies have shown it to damage DNA, kill human endothelial cells, and elicit both liver damage and allergic reactions.[10-14] The propylparaben found in Sara Lee® cinnamon rolls is a known endocrine disruptor that can mimic estrogen, and it is associated with breast cancer cells.[2,15-17] That sounds pretty scary. Those chemicals can't *really* be *that* bad, right? Surely the government has checked them for safety or they wouldn't be in our grocery stores, right?

Wrong.

**The U.S. government does not test these chemicals for safety.**[18] They don't even regulate or monitor them. So, who does? Who makes sure these chemicals are safe for us to eat? And, should we trust them to make those decisions? To answer those questions, we need to go back to the year 1958. That's the year our government made it legal to adulterate our food supply.

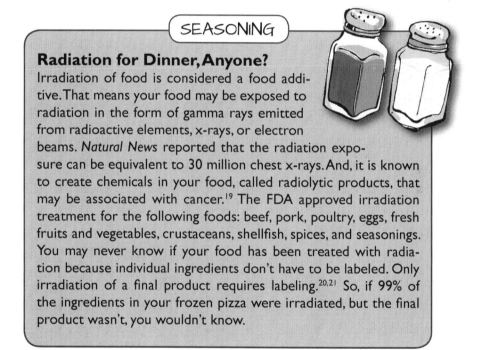

( SEASONING )

**Radiation for Dinner, Anyone?**
Irradiation of food is considered a food additive. That means your food may be exposed to radiation in the form of gamma rays emitted from radioactive elements, x-rays, or electron beams. *Natural News* reported that the radiation exposure can be equivalent to 30 million chest x-rays. And, it is known to create chemicals in your food, called radiolytic products, that may be associated with cancer.[19] The FDA approved irradiation treatment for the following foods: beef, pork, poultry, eggs, fresh fruits and vegetables, crustaceans, shellfish, spices, and seasonings. You may never know if your food has been treated with radiation because individual ingredients don't have to be labeled. Only irradiation of a final product requires labeling.[20,21] So, if 99% of the ingredients in your frozen pizza were irradiated, but the final product wasn't, you wouldn't know.

## Born Out Of Good Intention

Food additives are approved and regulated by the FDA. In 1958, President Eisenhower signed the Food Additive Amendment onto the Federal Food Drug and Cosmetic Act of 1938. With one stroke of a pen, the

FDA was given authority to decide which food additives could be used in our food supply and how they could be used.[22]

Under the new law, manufacturers were required to establish the safety of their own food additives and the FDA was given authority to check them for safety and oversee their use. Here's how it works: Industry submits their chemical additive for approval using a "food additive petition." Then, the FDA conducts an agency review of that chemical to determine if it is safe for us to eat. Part of that review involves a mandatory public notification and comment period to ensure the people are given a voice. "We the People" are entrusted, under this law, to be the watchdogs. A chemical is only supposed to be approved for use in our food after *both* the FDA and the people have the opportunity to review the information. After that entire process is complete, the FDA makes a final decision regarding the safety of the chemical and determines if it is allowed in our food supply.[3]

The original intent of the Food Additive Amendment was to make sure that the chemicals added to our food are safe for us to eat *before* we consumed them. That sounds like a common sense goal, but at the time the law was enacted, there were roughly 800 additives in our food supply and *nobody* was checking them for safety.[23] That was supposed to change with the passage of the Food Additive Amendment. Unfortunately, the implementation of the law has been a far cry from the original intent and it stems from a single loophole called the GRAS exemption.

( SEASONING )

## More Unconstitutional Laws!
"The Federal Food Drug and Cosmetic Act of 1938 is unconstitutional."[24]
"The 1958 Food Additive Amendment is unconstitutional."[24]

—Michael Farris, Constitutional attorney and Founder of Patrick Henry College in Virginia

Both laws are an over-reach of authority by the federal government. Both laws were imposed upon the American people through a distortion of the Commerce Clause (Article I, Section 8 of the Constitution of the United States).[24]

## Permission To Poison Our Food

The Food Additive Amendment contains what is commonly referred to as the GRAS exemption. The GRAS exemption was intended to be a good thing. It was designed to allow ingredients, such as oil and vinegar, to be added to foods without going through government "red tape".[23] The exempt chemicals are called GRAS or "generally recognized as safe." GRAS chemicals don't have to go through an FDA approval process before reaching supermarket shelves. They get a free pass.[25]

There are two paths for getting a chemical on the GRAS list. The first path is through initial date of use. According to the FDA, if an ingredient was used in our food supply *before* January 1, 1958 then it was determined to be GRAS "based on common use in food:"

> "Under sections 201(s) and 409 of the Act, and FDA's implementing regulations in 21 CFR 170.3 and 21 CFR 170.30, the use of a food substance may be GRAS either through scientific procedures or, for a substance used in food before 1958, through experience based on common use in food."[26]

That path to GRAS was supposed to include the types of ingredients your grandmother or great-grandmother had in her kitchen, such as: salt, spices, yeast, soybean oil, and water.[20] These types of commonly used ingredients didn't have to receive government approval since they were already widely used by 1958.[23] That sounds great! I applaud Congress for taking a common-sense approach to the law. They prevented ingredients like water and pepper from undergoing unnecessary and time-consuming safety tests. However, this path to GRAS exemption contains a fatal flaw.

The food supply was already adulterated by 1958. Yet, Congress chose that year as the default date, which implies they were okay with every chemical that was already in the food supply. Clearly they weren't, or the law wouldn't have been proposed in the first place. Besides, we know that Americans were already concerned about synthetic chemicals being added to their food. Since the early 1900s, Americans witnessed a new era of food as highly processed foods containing chemical additives popped up seemingly overnight. Oreos® and Crisco® appeared on grocery store shelves around the turn of the century. Velveeta®, Kool-Aid®, and Spam® followed close behind. Then, in the 1940s, the number of synthetic chemicals in our food supply increased dramatically.[27] Products such as Cheetos® hit the market, followed by Cheez Whiz®, Tang®, and TV dinners.

Scientists and citizens alike were leery of the chemicals being added to their food. In addition, the public's fear of getting cancer helped rally support behind stronger food laws.[28] So, when Congress delivered, why did they set the default GRAS date as the same year the law was passed? Why didn't they choose a date that marks the period before most of the newly invented processed "food stuffs" were created, like 1900? I don't know the answer, but I do know a consequence.

Trans fats.

Trans fats have been widely used since the 1950s, finding their way into doughnuts, cakes, biscuits, cookies, frozen pizza, and many other processed foods. If you've ever cooked with Crisco® or stick margarine, then you've eaten trans fats. These fats are artificial, meaning they are made by man and are, therefore, not found in nature. Trans fats are created in a laboratory by converting liquid vegetable oils into more solid fats, increasing their shelf life and making them less expensive than butter.[29] Interestingly, the two oils most commonly used to make trans fats are soybean and cottonseed. As we learned in chapter five, they happen to be two of the most subsidized crops in the U.S.[30]

In 1956, trans fats were already blamed for heart disease, primarily by a medical researcher named Ancel Keys (Remember that name. We will meet him again in chapter nine).[31] Yet, they still qualified for GRAS status because they were commonly used before the 1958 law came into effect.[30,32] As a result, Americans consumed trans fats for decades under the belief that the FDA determined they were safe. That's simply not the case. The FDA never tested trans fats for safety. They qualified for a free pass to the grocery store shelves because of the GRAS exemption. Recently, the FDA declared trans fats to be responsible for "eight deaths a day in the United States."[23] And, in 2015, largely because of a citizen petition, the FDA revoked the GRAS status of trans fats.[30,33] However, companies have 3 years to comply, so check your labels! You can find trans fats under the name "partially hydrogenated oils."[29]

Even though trans fats will be removed from our favorite baked goods and frozen meals, we still eat chemicals that made it onto the default GRAS list, and the FDA is still not checking them for safety. Even when new scientific research arises, the chemicals remain unchecked.[18] This path to GRAS is concerning, but it's not nearly as troubling as the second path.

## The Bad Apple

The second path for obtaining GRAS status is where our story gets interesting. Who decides which food additives are GRAS if an ingredient is introduced into our food supply after January 1, 1958?

I assumed it was the job of the FDA. After all, they are responsible for ensuring the safety of most of our food supply. Wouldn't they play a role in picking the chemicals that we eat on a *daily* basis?

Nope!

According to the Food Additive Amendment, it is *not* the job of the FDA to determine if a chemical is GRAS. They determine the safety and regulation of food additives, but not GRAS chemicals. Remember, GRAS means the chemical is *exempt* from food additive regulations. So, who has authority to determine GRAS status?

Nobody.

In a conversation over email, Steve Morris, Director of Food Safety and Agriculture at the Government Accountability Office (GAO), explained that Congress did not appoint anyone for that job. And, in the absence of leadership, industry stepped in:

> "Congress did not declare who would be responsible for determining substances to be GRAS in the 1958 Amendments to the Federal Food, Drug, and Cosmetic Act...In short, food manufacturers, for the purposes of marketing their products, determine whether an ingredient or substance to be added to food is GRAS."[34]

That means a company can use the exemption to bring their synthetic chemical ingredients directly from a laboratory to your dinner plate without FDA approval.[18]

This second path to GRAS is overwhelmingly used by industry.[22] "...over the past decade, almost all new chemicals added directly to food have gone through this GRAS exemption rather than the formal approval process intended by Congress," according to the Pew Charitable Trusts, a non-profit organization that exists to serve citizens.[3] In other words, the GRAS exemption has become a loophole for industry.

What does this mean for us, the consumer?

You can forget about knowing if chemicals are safe to eat *before* you eat them. Because of the GRAS exemption, we eat chemicals on a daily basis that have not been determined to be safe by the FDA. Let me say that again: **We currently eat chemicals in our food that the FDA has not determined to be safe.** That's a scary situation considering there are over 10,000 chemicals‡ added to our food supply.[3]

Included in that mix of 10,000 chemicals are the BHT and propylene glycol that I found lurking in the Pillsbury® bread mix. Both achieved GRAS status, which means that even though one is associated with cancer in animals and the other is used to de-ice airport runways, they are legally allowed in our foods without any safety checks, approval, or oversight from the FDA.[2,3,5,7,8] Propylparaben in Sara Lee® cinnamon rolls is associated with breast cancer cells, but it is GRAS.[2,15–17] It's not allowed in foods sold in the European Union, but it's apparently good enough for us in the United States.[35] And, if you think your pizza is safe to eat, think again. Some pizza sauces contain BHA, which is GRAS even though it is associated with behavioral issues including cognitive deficits.[36–38] But, it gets worse.

The National Toxicology Program lists BHA as "reasonably anticipated to be a human carcinogen," meaning it most likely causes cancer.[39] That organization is part of the U.S. Health and Human Services, which is the same organization that houses the FDA! So, our government knows BHA can cause cancer but they still allow it to be put in our food. How does it feel to be the guinea pig in a nation-wide chemical experiment?

## The Free Market Wins Again!

In 2015, General Mills Inc. released a statement promising to remove BHT from their cereals. According to the company website:

"We've heard BHT has kept some people from eating cereal, so we're removing it because we want more people to be able to enjoy our cereals."[40]

Currently, several of their cereals do not contain BHT including: Kix®, Lucky Charms®, Fiber One®, Cheerios®, and Reese's Puffs®.[40]

---

‡ For information on additional chemicals lurking in our foods, please refer to *Food Forensics* by Mike Adams.

## Bought And Paid For

Who is orchestrating this national chemical experiment?

"Experts."

All a company has to do to get their chemical on the GRAS list is have an "expert" declare it to be GRAS. So, who are these "experts" that determine which chemicals are safe for you and I to eat?[22]

In 2013, a study published in the *Journal of the American Medical Association* (JAMA) *Internal Medicine*, a premiere journal for medical doctors, revealed who these "experts" really are. According to the study, between 1997 and 2012, there were 451 new chemicals added to our food supply without FDA safety checks or oversight. The "experts" who verified the safety of these chemicals all had close ties to industry. They either had "a vested interest in the outcome of those assessments" or "relationships with manufacturers of food additives."[41] In other words, there was a clear conflict of interest.

These "experts" are frequently bought and paid for by industry. For instance, companies can use their own employees to declare their own chemical safe. They can also hire consultants. Either way, those "experts" are on the company payroll. To make matters worse, the safety determination process is often undisclosed, which means you and I don't have access to it.[23]

The demand for "experts" is so high that entire companies have been set up to farm them out to food companies who need someone to sign off on their food additives. Marion Nestle, Nutrition professor at New York University, went on record to reveal this new era of food regulation where "experts" are for hire:

> "The companies hire a consulting firm to get experts for them and then the experts review the information that's available and then they write a letter to FDA saying this additive should be considered GRAS...There are whole companies that are in the business of recruiting scientists to sign off on these things."[1]

As soon as one of these "experts" declares a chemical to be safe, the company can immediately add it to our food. There is no waiting period. They don't even have to notify the FDA! Notification is completely optional.[41] But wait, it gets worse.

Any company, domestic or foreign, can declare their own chemical to be GRAS. Who knows, a synthetic chemical made in a laboratory in China might be waiting for you in your next meal. But, don't worry. China also has "experts" that vouch for the safety of their chemicals.[18,42] I'm sure you have nothing to worry about. By the way, the FDA admits to not knowing which chemicals foreign countries are putting in our food. And, even if a foreign company did notify the FDA about their GRAS chemical, the FDA does not record or track the origin of chemicals. Consequently, they don't know how many chemicals we eat every day that originate from foreign countries.[18]

## Generally Recognized As Secret

The most important question for us, the consumers, is: Has the GRAS exemption compromised our food supply? Is our food less safe under the Food Additive amendment?

Yes!

Since companies don't have to notify the FDA of their GRAS determination, the FDA does not know which chemicals are in our food. It is estimated that roughly **1,000 chemicals have been added to our food without the FDA's knowledge**.[3] That's a frightening reality because the "FDA generally has no information about GRAS determinations that are not submitted to its notification program," according to the Government Accountability Office (GAO). Here's a simple question: If companies don't have to notify the FDA when they add chemicals to our food and some companies don't *voluntarily* provide the FDA with this information, how do we know what we are eating?

The answer is simple: We don't.

In 2013, the FDA Deputy Commissioner for Foods, Michael Taylor, admitted that the FDA is out of the loop when it comes to knowing which chemicals are put in our food supply. According to Mr. Taylor:

> "We're not driven by a sense that there is a pressing public health emergency. But there are decisions being made based on data that we don't have access to, and that creates a question about the basis on which those decisions are made."[3]

By the FDA's own admission, our food supply is adulterated right now, yet they don't consider it to be a "pressing public health emergency." I disagree. Studies are beginning to show a connection between chemicals in our food and disease. These chemicals may be contributing to the increase we see in food allergies, metabolic disorders, inflammatory diseases, and autoimmune conditions like multiple sclerosis.[43–46] And, since the FDA Deputy Commissioner of *Food* doesn't even know what chemical companies are putting in our food, I would say we have a problem. After all, if he doesn't know what we are eating, what are the odds of us finding out?

According to the Natural Resources Defense Council (NRDC), a non-profit watchdog group, the odds are close to zero:

> "It is often virtually impossible for the public to find out about the safety—or in many cases even the existence—of these chemicals in our food."[23]

The chance of us finding out which chemicals are in our food is so slim that the NRDC refers to the GRAS list as "generally recognized as *secret*."[23] Here's a question for you: How can you protect your health when you don't know what chemicals are in your food?

Oh, I forgot. We're not supposed to worry about that because the FDA is paid to do that job for us, right? How can the FDA be "protecting and promoting our health" if *they* don't even know what is in the food supply?

They simply can't. Yet, they seem okay with that. During a 2010 investigation, the GAO reported that, "FDA officials stated that companies making GRAS determinations without notifying the FDA were not a concern because the Federal Food, Drug, and Cosmetic Act makes companies, not FDA, responsible for GRAS determinations."[18] In other words, according to the FDA, it's not their job so they aren't concerned that our food supply is adulterated.

## Fox Guarding The Hen House

I had a difficult time believing that the FDA took a hands-off, unregulated approach to the GRAS list. Would the government voluntarily choose not to regulate such a big part of our food supply and, instead, hand that authority over to chemical companies?

To answer that question, I decided to find the GRAS database and analyze one of the company notifications for myself.

When a company voluntarily submits a GRAS notice to the FDA, it is listed on the FDA website in the GRAS database.§ One of the first chemicals listed was xylanase. It received GRAS status, which is concerning because xylanase is genetically engineered. And, according to the GRAS notice, Danisco® plans to put xylanase in our food, including: cereal, drinks, baked goods, and alcohol.

A thorough reading of the xylanase submission shows that Danisco® determined xylanase to be safe for us to eat based on scientific literature searches, a few studies that included eye and skin reaction experiments on rabbits, and a letter from an "expert."[49] The response from the FDA was "no questions," along with a letter stating the FDA acknowledges that DuPont™ (the parent company of Danisco®) has declared xylanase to be GRAS, but that the FDA itself has not determined this substance to be safe. But, don't take my word for it. The following statement was taken directly from the FDA letter addressed to DuPont® in response to the GRAS notification. It was signed by the Director of the Office of Food Additive Safety on May 7, 2015:

---

§ The GRAS Database can be found at: http://www.accessdata.fda.gov/scripts/fdcc/?set=SCOGS

"Based on the information provided by DuPont, as well as other information available to FDA, the agency has no questions at this time regarding DuPont's conclusion that xylanase enzyme preparation is GRAS under the intended conditions of use. The agency has not, however, made its own determination regarding the GRAS status of the subject use of xylanase enzyme preparation."[50]

There you have it: The FDA does not determine if chemicals are GRAS, nor do they affirm that chemicals deemed to be GRAS by industry are truly "generally recognized as safe." They simply state they don't have any questions.

The letter also reminded the manufacturer that the safety of their product is their own responsibility and not the responsibility of the FDA. That sounds crazy, but here it is in black and white:

"As always, it is the continuing responsibility of DuPont to ensure that food ingredients that the firm markets are safe, and are otherwise in compliance with all applicable legal and regulatory requirements."[50]

Consequently, xylanase is now on the GRAS list simply because the manufacturer claims it is safe. It's alarming to realize that a genetically engineered ingredient can be added to our food based on a letter from an "expert" and a few eye and skin tests on rabbits. Does that make you question the safety of the chemicals on the GRAS list?

*Natural News*, a citizen watch dog group, summed up the reality of the situation:

"...an overwhelming 99 percent of all food additives currently in use are either untested, were never submitted to the FDA at all or were submitted by industry insiders along with industry-funded safety data. In other words, **the fox is guarding the hen house** when it comes to food additive safety, as there is little-to-no credible oversight governing what millions of trusting Americans feed their families."[51] [emphasis added]

How did we get to a place where industry decides what is safe and the FDA doesn't even require a simple notification when chemicals are added to our foods? Was the system always like this? Has our food supply always been this ripe with adulteration? Surely the FDA could not have always been this hands-off.

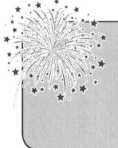

### The Free Market Wins Again!
Papa John's Pizza, Inc. removed 14 ingredients from their products in 2016, including artificial colors and some synthetic preservatives. As the third-largest pizza chain in America, Papa John's, Inc. is setting a new standard.[52]

## In The Dark From The Start

The lack of safety checks and oversight of chemicals in our food has existed from the start. The first GRAS list was published in 1958 and, initially, *nobody* evaluated it. Shockingly, the FDA admits that it "made no systematic attempt to evaluate available scientific information on the GRAS substances."[53] Instead of determining if the chemicals were safe, the FDA simply published a GRAS list. All of that changed when a GRAS substance was found to cause cancer.

In the 1960s, an artificial sweetener on the GRAS list, called cyclamate salts, came under fire because new scientific information revealed a connection between the artificial sweetener and cancer in rodents. Consequently, the FDA banned the sweetener.[18,54] That prompted President Richard Nixon to issue a White House directive in 1969 requiring the FDA to review *all* of the chemicals on the GRAS list to make sure they were safe.[55]

The FDA responded by hiring contractors to evaluate the safety of the GRAS ingredients, which led to the formation of a Select Committee on GRAS Substances (SCOGS). SCOGS was comprised of "experts" that were selected by the Life Sciences Research Office. According to the FDA, "By 1982, after 10 years of work, SCOGS had produced 151 detailed reports covering over 400 substances."[53] That sounds great, at first blush. Let's not forget that it took the FDA roughly 25 years to *partially* review the GRAS list *after* they had already published it. Plus, there were roughly 800 additives at the time the Food Additive Amendment was passed. SCOGUS evaluated roughly 400, so what happened with the evaluation of the other 400 or so chemicals?

According to the FDA, the safety report that was completed in 1982 "did not cover many substances that were marketed based on a manufacturer's independent conclusion that a use of a substance was GRAS."[53] Let's pause for a moment to consider the situation: The FDA admitted that "many" of the substances on the GRAS list were declared safe for us to eat based solely on the word of the companies that made those very same chemicals. That means there was no independent, third party analysis or government oversight of these chemicals. Keep in mind that we still eat some of these chemicals in our foods today.

Around the time the SCOGS review was taking place, the FDA changed their GRAS procedure. They created a *voluntary* "petition affirmation process," which began in 1972. Under this new procedure, companies still provided their own information to support a GRAS determination, including data from studies they funded themselves. But, the company could now ask the FDA to weigh in on whether or not a chemical was GRAS. As the FDA began receiving voluntary petitions, they "became aware of companies' independent GRAS determinations."[18] According to the GAO, companies had been deciding if their chemicals were GRAS without input from the FDA and the FDA didn't realize that until the petitions started pouring into their office.[18]

Interestingly, the petition affirmation process gave us our voice back. When companies utilize the GRAS loophole, there is no public notification or comment period required. The loophole shut us out of the approval process. However, under the petition affirmation process, the GRAS petitions were published in the Federal Register and a public comment period was required before a final ruling was issued by the FDA.[18]

It wouldn't be long before our voices were silenced again, or at least muffled. By the 1990's, chemicals were flooding the market and the FDA could not keep up with the petitions. So, the FDA changed the GRAS rule again "to enable the agency to use its resources more efficiently and effectively."[53] In 1997, citing limited resources, the *voluntary* "notification procedure" was launched.[23] This new *voluntary* procedure marked a fundamental shift in GRAS policy. **The public comment period was removed, effectively silencing us.** In addition, the FDA would no longer "affirm" a chemical was GRAS.[18] Instead, the FDA would simply post a response on their website with 3 possible outcomes:

1. "FDA has no questions about the notifier's conclusion of GRAS status.
2. The notice does not provide a basis for a conclusion of GRAS status.
3. At the notifier's request, FDA ceased to evaluate the notice."[53]

Receiving a "no questions" response is like finding the golden ticket! It means the FDA does not question the GRAS determination made by a company. Remember xylanase? It received a "no questions" response, which gave it a free pass to be added to our foods with no regulations or oversight. A "no questions" response does *not* mean the FDA agrees that xylanase is GRAS. They just don't question the company's conclusion. In other words, the **FDA does not approve any chemicals on the GRAS list.**

I contend that the GRAS list perpetuates the veil of unearned trust in the food supply by providing Americans with a false sense of security about their food. The mere act of having a list of chemicals that are "generally recognized as safe" gives consumers the impression that the FDA has evaluated and approved those chemicals for us to eat. Additionally,

---

( SEASONING )

### Birth of the Food Additive Amendment

The 1906 Pure Food and Drugs Act turned out to be a pit bull with no teeth. In 1933, the FDA called the law "obsolete" and recommended a "complete revision."[28] A five-year legislative battle ensued. Then, 107 people, including several children, died from consuming a drug called "Elixir of Sulfanilamide" in 1937. The drug itself didn't kill them; a poisonous additive was to blame. It was the solvent known as diethylene glycol. The tragedy rallied public support behind stronger drug and food laws. Less than one year later, Congress passed the Federal Food, Drug, and Cosmetics (FDC) Act of 1938. Among other provisions, this new law authorized factory inspections, standards of identity for foods, and required safe tolerances to be set for "unavoidable poisonous substances."[28] The Food Additive Amendment, containing the GRAS exemption, was amended to this law in 1958.

---

HANDS OFF MY FOOD!

the GRAS list implies that only those chemicals, and no others, are added to the foods we buy. That's clearly not true. The truth is that the FDA doesn't test the chemicals we eat to determine if they are safe. They don't even give their opinion on whether or not a chemical is safe. They simply respond with "no questions."

## FDA Relinquishes Control

According to the FDA, preventing food adulteration is its job. Therefore, it's our duty to ask if the FDA has taken any steps towards resolving the adulteration problem with chemical additives. In other words, is the FDA doing its job?

Historically, the FDA has taken a reactionary approach to the GRAS list. The Pew Charitable Trust hired a team of scientists and lawyers to analyze the Food Additive program. They found that the FDA checks the safety of a chemical only *after* a problem arises or when the company asks for a check:

> "FDA has not reevaluated the safety of many chemicals originally approved decades ago, generally rechecking safety only when requested by a company to do so, or when presented with allegations of serious adverse health effects."[3]

The FDA has authority to de-GRAS or ban a chemical if it has resulted in adverse health effects. They've banned chemicals before but, according to a 2010 GAO investigation, the FDA "has not systematically reconsidered GRAS substances since the 1980s."[18] Even as new scientific information has emerged, the safety of chemicals on the GRAS list has not been reassessed.

The FDA's reactionary approach to the GRAS list is sometimes blamed on its limited authority. Remember, according to the original Act, the FDA "is not required to review substances…added to food that are generally recognized as safe (GRAS)."[18] However, according to the GAO, the FDA not only has authority to de-GRAS a chemical, it can affirm a chemical is GRAS:

> "FDA, on its own initiative, may affirm in regulation that a substance, when used as indicated, is regarded by the Commissioner as GRAS. Alternatively, FDA may issue a regulation prohibiting a substance if the Commissioner determines, among other

things, it has not been shown by adequate scientific data to be safe for use in human food."[34]

In addition, the FDA has authority to monitor companies to make sure their GRAS determinations have been conducted properly, but it doesn't. In 1997, the FDA said it would conduct random audits of companies, but it didn't. The FDA also has authority to issue guidance on what constitutes an "expert," including what constitutes a conflict of interest for these "experts," but it hasn't.[18]

The FDA has taken such a lackadaisical approach to the GRAS list that the 2010 GAO investigation concluded:

> "FDA oversight process does not help ensure the safety of all new GRAS determinations…FDA is not systematically ensuring the continued safety of current GRAS substances."[18]

In fact, it took almost 20 years for the FDA to decide if the *voluntary* GRAS "notification procedure" would stick around. The FDA began testing that procedure in 1997. The final ruling was issued in 2016 (effective October 17, 2016).[56] Why did it take nearly 20 years to issue a ruling?

According to the FDA, they were in no hurry. During a 2010 GAO investigation, FDA officials told the GAO, "[T]he agency has higher priorities and currently has no specific schedule for doing so." In addition, FDA officials reported that, "the program has been operating effectively under the proposed rule."[18]

To its credit, the FDA has issued guidelines to industry regarding how to verify the safety of chemical additives. Unfortunately, according to the PEW Charitable Trusts, these guidelines rely on "outdated science" that "has not been significantly updated for decades."[3] They don't even include critical questions regarding food safety, such as:

- Does the additive impact human behavior?
- Does the additive disrupt hormonal balance?
- How does the additive affect sensitive populations?

In addition, according to the outdated FDA guidelines, industry does not have to demonstrate how their chemical additive is processed and eliminated by the body. That's a problem. Without knowing how the chemical moves through your body, industry doesn't know which organs to target for safety testing. In addition, how does industry know the chemical does not accumulate in fat tissue or damage organs if they don't even know where to look for it? These are some of the same concerns that were raised by the Select Committee on GRAS Substances (SCOGUS) over 30 years ago. They "remain unresolved and relevant today."[3]

In addition to outdated industry guidelines, the FDA cannot ensure these chemicals are safe for us to eat because it doesn't know our overall exposure. Companies don't have to tell the FDA how much of a GRAS chemical they are putting in our food. Additionally, if we are exposed to a chemical through our food and the environment, sometimes both the FDA and the Environmental Protection Agency (EPA) regulate that chemical. When this occurs, the two agencies don't talk to each other. Therefore, the FDA cannot accurately assess our cumulative exposure to these chemicals. **There is no way for the FDA to know how much of each chemical we are exposed to on a daily basis.**[3]

The FDA knows that statement is true. In 2014, the FDA acknowledged that we have a problem with food adulteration in our country and that it stems from the GRAS list:

> "We have seen a growth in the marketplace of beverages and other conventional foods that contain novel substances, such as added botanical ingredients or their extracts. Some of these substances have not previously been used in conventional foods and may be unapproved food additives. Other substances that have been present in the food supply for many years are now being added to beverages and other conventional foods at levels in excess of their traditional use levels, or in new beverages or other conventional foods. This trend raises questions regarding whether these new uses are unapproved food additive uses."[25] [emphasis added]

Food adulteration was the reason the FDA came into existence in 1906. Preventing food adulteration was declared to be *the job* of the FDA. Now the agency is admitting there is a problem. So, how is the FDA currently handling the food adulteration resulting from the GRAS list?

The FDA released a document titled, "Guidance for Industry: Considerations regarding substances added to foods, including beverages and dietary substances." The document contains *voluntary* and "nonbinding recommendations" for industry including: a reminder that industry is responsible for ensuring the safety of their own products and their own compliance with the laws. According to the FDA:

> "It is your responsibility to ensure that substances added to foods you manufacture or distribute, including non-dietary ingredients in dietary supplements, comply with all applicable regulatory requirements for substances added to food."[25]

That's the GRAS loophole in action. Not only can these chemical companies add ingredients to their products without getting approval, they are legally allowed to regulate themselves with no binding guidelines from government. Interestingly, the U.S. is the only developed country in the world that allows chemical additives in their food supply without government approval. No other developed country does this. They all require government approval *before* chemicals are released into their food.[3] That was the intention of the Food Additive Amendment. Clearly, we've missed the mark.

Why would we expect anything different from the FDA, considering it has consistently taken a lackadaisical approach to overseeing chemical additives since the 1958 law was passed? Remember, the FDA had to be ordered by President Nixon to review the GRAS list for safety. Even after a Presidential directive was issued, the FDA only did half the job. And, it out-sourced it! In the midst of a leadership vacuum, companies saw the advantage and took it. It's a case of survival of the fittest. Industry won and consumers lost. By their own admission, the FDA chooses not to regulate or monitor GRAS chemicals. It is an active participant in the loophole. In fact, the FDA increased the size of the GRAS list by making "spices, seasonings, and flavorings" eligible for GRAS status.[18] It opened the floodgates for thousands of flavorings to enter the marketplace. The flavor industry had a field day with that ruling.

## While The Parents Are Away

Flavors make up the largest portion of the GRAS list. Check the ingredient labels of your favorite foods and you'll likely find the words "artificial flavor" or "natural flavor." Even organic foods can contain "natural flavor." Why do so many of our foods contain flavoring?

Food manufacturers use so many flavorings because when whole foods are processed, the flavors are often destroyed. Manufacturers add flavors back to our foods to make them taste good again, except those flavorings are made in a laboratory. For instance, acetaldehyde is a GRAS-approved flavoring. It is a flammable liquid that was designated as a carcinogen by the International Agency for Research on Cancer.[59] Does that sound like a chemical you want to eat?

Do you know which chemicals are used to make the "artificial" or "natural" flavoring in *your* favorite treat?

You and I will probably never know the answer to that question because companies are not required to list those ingredients on the food label. The chemicals used to create the flavors we love, like Cool Ranch Doritos® and Chocolate Mint Crème Oreos®, are considered industry trade secrets. We do know, however, that when scientists create a flavor, they often use a long list of chemical ingredients. In fact, more than 100 different chemicals can be used to create just one flavor![60] According to Mitchell Cheeseman, former director of the FDA's Office of Food Additive Safety, if companies had to list the chemical names of flavorings, "the label would be substantially longer than it is for most foods."[55]

If companies won't tell us which chemicals make up flavorings, and the FDA doesn't mandate transparency, can we trust them? Who determines if flavorings are safe for us to eat?

The leadership vacuum that was created by the FDA's hands-off approach to flavorings gave rise to an industry solution. Beginning in 1959, a new generation of GRAS ingredients was born with the formation of the Flavor and Extract Manufacturers Association (FEMA).[61] FEMA sidestepped the government almost entirely by creating its own GRAS determination process. FEMA has determined over 2,600 substances to be GRAS since 1960. In comparison, 274 chemicals have gone through the FDA's voluntary GRAS Notification Program since 1998.[18]

FEMA consists of roughly 120 member companies. These companies submit GRAS applications to FEMA's "expert" panel instead of going through the FDA notification process.[18] Once approved, FEMA notifies the FDA of their GRAS determinations. At first glance, FEMA sounds pretty great. After all, it's a third-party trade organization that independently certifies a GRAS list. What could go wrong?

In the absence of guidance documents from the FDA, industry must create their own guidelines. That's exactly what FEMA has done when determining if a chemical may cause cancer. FEMA's attorney and senior science advisor stated that, "Whether a food ingredient is GRAS depends on general recognition of safety, not on safety *per se*...a substance that causes tumors in laboratory animals at high doses is nevertheless GRAS under conditions of intended use in human food..."[61] The problem with FEMA's criteria is that it might be illegal. According to the Food Additives Amendment of 1958, "...no additive shall be deemed to be safe if it is found to induce cancer when ingested by man or animal..."[22] Has FEMA approved chemicals for us to eat that have been shown to induce cancer in animals?

Yes!

FEMA determined isoeugenol to be GRAS even though a 2-year study conducted by the National Toxicology Program determined isoeugenol to be carcinogenic in rats. The scientists concluded, "There was clear evidence of carcinogenic activity of isoeugenol..."[62] Just to be clear: the National Toxicology Program is part of the U.S. Department of Health and Human Services. This is the same Health and Human Services that houses the FDA. That means our government is saying that isoeugenol is carcinogenic but FEMA is saying it's safe for us to eat.

FEMA defended their position on isoeugenol by claiming that the cancer reported in the 2-year study "is not relevant to humans who consume isoeugenol at low non-toxic levels (<0.1 mg/kg bw per day)."[63] In other words, FEMA acknowledges that isoeugenol can cause cancer but declared it safe for humans based on the assumption that we eat small enough quantities to not cause a problem. Consequently, isoeugenol made the GRAS list. But, how does FEMA know we only eat small quantities of isoeugenol when the FDA doesn't track the GRAS chemicals?

According to the National Cancer Institute, there is "widespread human exposure" to this chemical.[62] Thanks to FEMA, it can be found in baked goods, chewing gum, and non-alcoholic drinks.[62] Check your food labels!

## The Free Market Wins Again!

In 2015, General Mills Inc. pledged to remove artificial flavors and artificial colors from their cereals. Why? Consumer demand. According to General Mills Inc.:

"Our cereal team is always listening to consumers about how we can improve our cereals and make them better. In recent years, we've heard that artificial ingredients aren't what you are looking for in your bowl. So today, we've announced that we are committing to remove artificial flavors and colors from artificial sources from the rest of General Mills cereals."[64]

## Proof Is In The Pudding

At least isoeugenol was tested on rats before it was released into our food supply. According to a 2013 study released by The Pew Charitable Trusts, most chemicals added to our food are not even tested on lab rats before they are sold to us for consumption:

"Our investigation found that most additives are not tested for safety in accordance with FDA's limited testing recommendations. Agency guidelines, for example, say that chemicals intentionally added to food should be fed to laboratory animals to identify potential harmful effects, but we found that in the majority of cases, chemicals directly added to food did not undergo this very basic test…And when health and safety studies indicate possible problems, food companies are not obligated to notify the agency except in very limited circumstances."[3]

How do you feel about eating propylparaben in your Sara Lee® cinnamon rolls or propyl gallate in your Pop Secret® popcorn, knowing that these chemicals may not have undergone safety testing?[23] Even if they were tested for safety, "many companies' GRAS safety determinations are seriously flawed," according to the Pew Charitable Trusts.[3] In addition, "Companies sometimes make safety decisions with little understanding of the law or the science," according to an investigative report by the NRDC.[23] They found documented cases where companies approved their chemical for use in our food even though it was known to cause potentially serious allergic reactions or interactions with common drugs. In addition, some companies planned to use larger quantities of the chemical than what was determined to be safe.[23]

The quality of GRAS notices have been so poor that when the FDA is asked by a manufacturer to review a GRAS determination, the FDA "rejects or triggers withdrawal of about one in five notices."[23] Thus, 20% of the notices that manufacturer's *voluntarily* submitted to the FDA were rejected or withdrawn. You don't want to get a rejection notice because the FDA publishes the safety concerns on their website for everyone to see.[23] But, that's not the case when a notice is withdrawn.

Through a Freedom of Information request, the NRDC was able to identify a handful of GRAS notifications that were voluntarily submitted to the FDA and then withdrawn by the company. Why would a company go through the trouble of submitting a packet of information only to withdraw it?

Unlike rejections, the FDA publishes withdrawals on their website *without* indicating any safety concerns that prompted the withdrawal. It turns out that if a submission is on track to be rejected, the FDA will sometimes give the company a chance to withdraw the submission, according to the NRDC.[23] Talk about a cozy relationship between industry and government!

Let's take a look at what happens when a notification is withdrawn. Epigallocatechin-3-gallate (EGCG) was imported to the U.S. for use in juices, sports drinks, soft drinks, and bottled teas. But, it may cause leukemia in unborn babies.[65] Furthermore, EGCG was shown to harm the liver, thyroid, testis, and gastrointestinal tract in a short-term rat study.[23] It can also have a potentially dangerous interaction with sodium nitrite (a common preservative) and acetaminophen (found in Tylenol).[65] Based on this knowledge, do you think the FDA banned this chemical from our food supply?

The FDA did not ban EGCG.

The manufacturer tried to get EGCG on the GRAS list, but they withdrew their notification. Hence, EGCG is not on the GRAS list and the FDA did not approve it for use in our food supply. However, the NRDC found EGCG in more than 25 food products sold in the U.S.[23] How does a product that didn't make the GRAS list and has not been approved by the FDA end up on our grocery store shelves?

The NRDC wondered the same thing. After gaining access to FDA records through a Freedom of Information request, the NRDC found out that if a company withdraws their GRAS notification, "The withdrawal does not prevent the company from continuing to market the product for use in food."[23] In other words, a company can withdrawal their GRAS notice and still put their product on the market.[23]

Sadly, EGCG was not an anomaly:

- A Japanese company wanted to put a neurotransmitter called Gamma-aminobutyric acid (GABA) in our beverages, gum, coffee, tea, and candy. GABA is reported to elicit a calming effect by inhibiting nerve transmissions in the brain. The company submitted a GRAS notice to the FDA with product specifications in Japanese. Additionally, they wanted to add more neurotransmitter to our foods than what the company considered to be a safe exposure level. The GRAS notice was withdrawn. The Japanese company told the NRDC that they are adding GABA to dietary supplements sold in the U.S., but they are not adding it to our foods. Yet, the NRDC found five foods sold in the U.S. that contain this neurotransmitter.[23]
- An Australian company declared sweet lupin protein, fiber, and flour to be GRAS. They wanted to add these chemicals to our baked goods. There was only one problem: These chemicals can cause an allergic reaction if you have a peanut allergy. The FDA did not believe that a product-warning label was enough. The GRAS notice was withdrawn. Yet, sweet lupin was found by the FRDC in over 20 food products and none had a warning label.[23]

- Theobromine was declared GRAS by a U.S. company that wanted to market this chemical in our cereal, bread, candy, yogurt, drinks, and chewing gum. It is used as a diuretic, vasodilator, and heart stimulant.[66] Theobromine was reported to delay bone formation in rats and resulted in testicular degeneration in both rats and rabbits. Additionally, the company wanted to feed us five times the level that was considered safe by the company's own consultant. They also planned to put this chemical in baby food. Their GRAS notice was withdrawn. But the NRDC found theobromine in more than 20 food products sold in the U.S.[23]

Given these examples of chemicals that were voluntarily submitted to the FDA for review, I wonder about the quality of the GRAS determinations that were *not* submitted to the FDA for review.

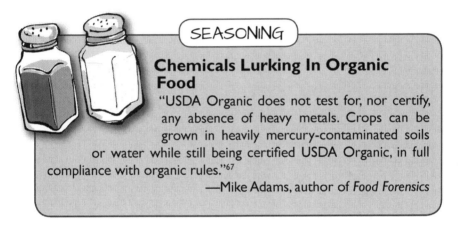

## SEASONING

### Chemicals Lurking In Organic Food

"USDA Organic does not test for, nor certify, any absence of heavy metals. Crops can be grown in heavily mercury-contaminated soils or water while still being certified USDA Organic, in full compliance with organic rules."[67]

—Mike Adams, author of *Food Forensics*

## Incentivizing Business

It's easy to blame companies for utilizing the GRAS loophole. But remember, companies operate on incentive, just like we do. And, there are incentives for choosing the GRAS path over the food additive path:

1. **GRAS carries weight in industry.** After working in the supplement industry, I can tell you that it's a big deal to make it on the GRAS list. When I helped formulate supplements and analyze ingredients from prospective suppliers, we would not touch the product unless it was GRAS. It's like a right of passage in the world of industry. There was even a saying where I worked, "If

it's not GRAS, it doesn't pass." Sadly, at the time, I did not know the truth about the GRAS list. I thought it was the governments' list of safe ingredients that were verified and tested by the FDA. That's the veil in action-Scientists assuming GRAS means "safe" and then adding those ingredients to our foods. Regardless, companies are incentivized to make the GRAS list.

2. **The short-term gains outweigh the long-term risks.** The chemical additives in our foods are added in small quantities. Therefore, they are unlikely to cause an **acute** health problem. Let's give industry some credit: We don't see people keeling over from an acute reaction to a food additive. Even when I worked for supplement companies, we performed acute testing on products. We often consumed the products ourselves.

The problem lies with the **long-term** health consequences. **There is no long-term safety or toxicity testing of GRAS chemicals.** That's concerning because these chemicals are more likely to cause health problems years down the road due to continual, small-dose exposure.[23] However, if you developed cancer from consuming one of these chemicals, how could you prove the cause was a single chemical when there are over 10,000 chemicals in our food supply?

From that perspective, adding a single chemical to a food doesn't seem like such a risky business decision. Besides, if the FDA doesn't even know that a company is putting a chemical in our food, how are they going to hold that company accountable for any health effects, whether immediate or long-term? According to The Pew Charitable Trusts:

> "If one of these chemicals was causing health problems short of immediate serious injury, it is unlikely that FDA would detect the problem unless the food industry alerted the agency."[3]

Proving actual harm from a chemical additive is like finding a needle in a haystack as tall as a New York skyscraper. Even the FDA admitted that our legal system does not hold companies accountable for food adulteration because it's too difficult to determine liability:

"Currently, the legal system does not ensure the optimum level of safety for foods because consumers who become ill often do not know the reason for, or source of, their illness. Even in cases where consumers are aware that their illness was contracted from a specific food, it is often difficult to determine who is ultimately responsible for their illness, since the particular source of contamination is not known in many circumstances."[68]

One reason the source of illness from a food is often unknown is because there is **no FDA labeling requirement.** The manufacturer is under no obligation to tell us whether or not the FDA has reviewed the chemical they added to our food. According to the NRDC, "There are no warning labels. There is no disclosure. As a consequence, they [the consumer] may unknowingly be putting their health at risk."[23]

3. **GRAS utilizes fewer resources.** According to Pew's research, "The food industry (and, to some extent, the agency itself) relies on the GRAS exemption because it believes that the food additive petition process that Congress adopted in 1958 is too burdensome and time-consuming, requiring that FDA use extensive formal rulemaking procedures. It prefers the GRAS notification program because it is informal and, as currently constructed, is voluntary."[3]

   If you owned a company, would you choose to deal with the government paperwork and expense that comes with the food additive process, or would you opt for a voluntary process that is overseen by your own company?

It's important to remember that using the GRAS loophole may be morally questionable, but it's not illegal. Companies are legally allowed to declare their products as GRAS. For that matter, the FDA is also following the rules. So, what's the *real* problem?

## We Let It Happen

When I learned about our government watchdog abdicating responsibility, and industry putting short-term profits ahead of our long-term health, I was ready to pounce! The government is supposed to be

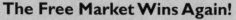

## The Free Market Wins Again!

As of 2016, Kraft Macaroni & Cheese® no longer contains artificial preservatives or synthetic dyes.[69] According to Kraft's® website:

"When parents talk, we listen. We know you want to feel good about what you eat and serve your family. This includes everything from improved nutrition to simpler ingredients. You told us you wanted to incorporate more foods with protein, calcium and whole grains into your diets and with no artificial flavors, preservatives or dyes. We heard you."[70]

Kraft® removed all dyes, artificial flavors, and artificial preservatives from all varieties of Kraft Macaroni & Cheese® in 2016.[70] The synthetic dyes were replaced with natural ingredients, like paprika and turmeric.[69]

"protecting and promoting" our health, and industry relies on consumers to stay in business. How could they not look out for our best interest? But, then I realized: I'm complicit too.

It's not a priority for industry to spend money on safety measures as long as the market doesn't place that demand on the company. You can blame the company, but is that really the problem? What drives a company?

Profits.

A company cannot exist without profit. We cannot expect companies to cut into their profits when there is no demand. Companies respond to *our* demand. If they don't, they may eventually go out of business. Think about this: Companies are responding right now to our lack of demand. In other words, **we are not demanding safety when we choose our food**; therefore, companies have no incentive to invest in safety measures.

Even the FDA agrees that consumers need to place demand on companies to ensure the safety of the chemicals in our food supply:

"…the lack of awareness and information about the [safety] risks suggests than an inefficiently low demand may exist for food products that are produced using adequate measures to prevent foodborne illness, adulteration, or contamination. Because the demand for many manufactured or processed foods may not be sufficiently affected by safety considerations, incentives to invest in safety measures from farm to fork is diminished. Consequently, the market may not provide the incentives necessary for optimal food safety."[68]

**The FDA sees us, the consumer, as the solution.** They're right! We can make our food safer by placing demand on companies. The first step is to be aware of what you are eating. Do you read your food labels? Or, do you blindly trust what is sold in the supermarkets and restaurants?

The most effective way to change the system is to change our behavior and let the market respond. That requires us to read our food labels, and act on that information.

## What You Can Do

You can petition the FDA to change a regulatory process. It's called a citizen petition.[18] But, I wouldn't hold your breath waiting for a response. Over 30 organizations filed comments regarding the 1997 GRAS notification process. It took nearly 20 years for the FDA to respond.[56] And, remember how I told you that the FDA removed trans fats from the GRAS list? The ruling came only after a citizen sued the FDA for not responding to his citizen petition.[32]

Our best bet is to speak with our dollars and make companies speak with theirs:

- **At the grocery store:**
  - Buy preservative-free chips, crackers, and cookies. Look for the words "no preservatives" or "preservative free" on the food label.
  - Buy processed foods that do not contain artificial or natural flavor. Look for the words "no artificial flavoring" on the food label. In addition, if the ingredient list contains the words "artificial flavor" or "natural flavor," don't buy the product.
  - Instead of buying pre-made desserts containing untested chemical additives, try baking from scratch. Recipes, as well as a cookbook filled with my son's favorite treats, can be found at: www.handsoffmyfood.com
- **When eating out:**
  - The next time you eat at a restaurant or fast-food chain, ask to see the ingredient list for the food you are about to order.

Knowing what's in your food before you decide to eat it provides the opportunity to make conscious decisions, as opposed to blindly trusting the food supply.

o Choose restaurants that are making an effort to remove untested chemicals from their menu, including: Chipotle, Elevation Burger, Panera, Pizza Fusion, Papa John's, Jason's deli, and Veggie Grill.

- **In your pantry:** When I started looking for untested chemicals on my food labels, it seemed like everything in my pantry was adulterated with synthetic and untested chemicals. So, let's take it one step at a time. If you feel inclined, go to your kitchen and check your favorite processed food to see if it contains either 'natural' or 'artificial' flavorings. If it does, you have options:

o Stop eating that product. Once you stop buying the product, the company loses profits. When enough of us stop buying that product, the company will conduct a focus group to determine why the demand decreased. Then, they will change their formulation. To help move the market:

➢ Call or email the company to report why you have stopped eating their product. You can also tell them you will not eat the product until the offending chemical is removed.

➢ Ask your friends and family to join you in putting pressure on the company.

➢ Start an online petition to get that chemical removed from your favorite food. Starting a petition can be free using websites such as: www.change.org or www.care2.com

o If you just can't live without your favorite processed food, call the manufacturer and demand a full list of the chemical names that are in that product, including the list of chemicals used to create the flavoring. If they provide that information, read the list and decide if you still want to eat those chemicals. If they don't reveal the ingredient list then you can decide if you trust the company or if you prefer to stop eating that food. Either way, you'll have made an informed decision.

o Eat less of that food. By decreasing demand for that product, you help move the market.

## Take Home Message

Congress passed the Food Additive Amendment in 1958 to put watchdogs in place that would oversee the chemicals being added to our foods. You and I, along with the FDA, are those watchdogs. Unfortunately, the law had the opposite effect. It created the GRAS loophole, which allows companies to decide which synthetic chemicals are in our foods and how much of each chemical we are exposed to. Consequently, most of us eat synthetic chemicals every day that are neither safety tested nor regulated by the FDA.

The law also helped perpetuate the unearned veil of trust. By creating a GRAS list, consumers may have been led to believe that the FDA approved those chemicals and regulates their use. Consequently, we have relinquished our duty as watchdogs over both industry and the FDA. In doing so, we expose ourselves to potential long-term health problems stemming from our cumulative exposure to unknown levels of synthetic chemicals in our food.

The government admits our food supply is in trouble, but what are they doing about it? They defer to the consumer. And, they're right! It's time to reclaim our voice. Instead of throwing money at the problem by giving the FDA more of our tax dollars to fix a problem they clearly don't think is their job, why don't we try a different approach?

You and I can fix this problem. Only we can move the market. It all begins with reading our food labels.

## Moving Forward

Next, we'll learn about the genetically modified hormone that makes cows sick, resulting in pus, blood, and bacteria in our milk. But first, let's take a short break and grab a snack. I recommend a sandwich made with Wonder® Bread and a cold glass of Kool-Aid® to wash it down. You'll be sure to get your daily recommendation of GRAS chemicals, including a hefty serving of propionate, vegetable monoglycerides, artificial and natural flavoring, and BHA, which is likely carcinogenic.[39,71] But, I'm sure these chemicals are safe to eat. After all, they're on the GRAS list. Surely *someone* has checked them for safety. Bon appetite!

CHAPTER 7:

# rBGH

## *The Milk Label That Sparked A Revolution*

This is the story that lifted my veil of unearned trust. It all started with a simple act: I read my milk label.

One day I noticed something unusual on my milk label. I had never noticed it before. It was a statement that read:

"According to the FDA, there is no significant difference in milk from rBGH treated cows and non-rBGH treated cows. FDA has determined that food products from cows treated with rBGH are safe for human consumption."

When I read that disclaimer, a red flag raised in my mind. Have you ever had one of those moments when your gut tells you that something is wrong? Every fiber of my being knew there was more to that 2-sentence label. Someone was hiding something. I put down my gallon of milk and headed straight to my computer.

A quick Internet search revealed that rBGH is a genetically engineered hormone given to dairy cows. I found news stories that seemed outrageous, including one claiming babies and young boys grew breasts because they drank milk from cows that were treated with rBGH. For example, in 2011 an article published by the *Huffington Post* reported that female infants in China grew breasts because their formula contained rBGH. The babies were only 4-15 months old and they already had estrogen levels as high as an adult woman.[1] That story sounded sensationalized, so I switched my focus from news articles to the scientific literature. That's when my concern grew rapidly.

Among the scientific literature were numerous studies[†] supporting a connection between rBGH and some cancers, including:

- **Colon cancer**[2–11]
- **Breast cancer**[4,12–30]
- **Childhood cancers**[31,32]
- **Prostate cancer**[33–39]

Does a connection between rBGH and cancer mean that rBGH definitively causes cancer?

No.

Honest scientists will tell you that we cannot *prove* anything because we cannot definitively determine cause and effect. We can never truly isolate one factor because there are so many caveats when looking at data pertaining to humans, such as: what they eat, their unique genetic makeup, if they live near power lines, etc. Hence, scientists cannot determine that rBGH will give you cancer. They can only report associations.

As I poured over the scientific literature, I concluded that an association exists between rBGH and cancer. From my analysis of the data, that relationship is strong enough to warrant not serving rBGH milk to my family. So, I spent the next hour reading every product label in my kitchen. I looked for the FDA disclaimer and any statement from the manufacturer indicating the product did not contain rBGH. I was crushed to find out that my older son's favorite ice cream contained rBGH. I personally approved that ice cream for my son to eat. It's "100% natural" and made from cream. It does not contain artificial sugar, sweetener, coloring, flavoring, preservatives, additives, or carrageenan. However, nowhere on the label does it mention anything about being free of rBGH. The label does boast about the company being "partially powered by wind." So, they are hurting our children, but saving the planet in the process.

---

† For a more detailed analysis of the association between rBGH and cancer, I recommend reading Dr. Samuel Epstein's book titled, *What's In Your Milk*. Dr. Epstein is the Chairman of the international Cancer Prevention Coalition.

My oldest son had consumed that "healthy" ice cream for nearly a year. How did this happen? How did I not know about rBGH? I needed answers. So, I continued to investigate.

I learned that the United States is one of the only modernized countries to allow the use of rBGH in dairy cows. **Canada, Japan, Australia, New Zealand, and the European Union (made up of 28 countries) banned rBGH.**[40,41] Think about that: Other countries won't allow their citizens to drink our milk but, according to the FDA, it's good enough for Americans.

In fact, up to one-third of dairy cows in the U.S. are treated with rBGH.[41,42] It's primarily used by large factory farmers.[43] These are the same farmers who supply most of the grocery stores with milk, which means **most of us have been exposed to rBGH at some point.**

Any of your dairy products might contain milk that came from rBGH treated cows, including: milk, cheese, butter, and ice cream. In addition, milk or milk components are frequently used in processed foods. That's concerning since roughly 75% of the American diet consists of processed foods.[44] How many of those processed foods do you think contain milk components from cows treated with rBGH?

We may never know. You can check your food label. It *might* indicate if the milk came from cows treated with rBGH. But, it doesn't have to. Labeling food products that contain milk from rBGH-treated cows is not mandatory.[45]

Why is rBGH in our milk any ways? And, why is there such a disconnect between the scientific evidence against rBGH and the FDA's stance that rBGH is perfectly safe?

It didn't add up. After all, if the FDA is right and rBGH milk is the same as regular milk then why did other countries ban it? To answer those questions, I needed to see the evidence for myself. I needed to figure out what rBGH does in our bodies and how it got approved.

## What Is rBGH?

rBGH is a genetically engineered hormone. It is called recombinant Bovine Growth Hormone or rBGH for short. It is also called somatotropin (rbST).

## How Is rBGH Made?

rBGH is created in a lab by combining cow genes with genes from bacteria. It sounds crazy, but it's true. Scientists take a cow gene and insert it into the bacteria *E. Coli*. Once the cow gene is added to the *E. Coli* gene, the new genetically engineered *E. Coli* bacteria makes a new hormone known as recombinant bovine growth hormone (rBGH). This hormone is then injected into the cow.[46,47]

I used to think of genetic engineering as a precise scientific process that is highly controlled by scientists in the laboratory. It's not. In reality, it's a messy process. For instance, when scientists want to add genes to a new organism, one method they use is a "gene gun." Scientists load the gun with the gene pieces and shoot them into a bowl of DNA. The goal is to get some of the genes in the right place. Does that sound precise to you?

My point is that the process of engineering genes is complicated and has unintended consequences. Before we insert these genes into our food supply, we should make sure we understand both the intended and unintended consequences.

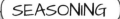

### SEASONING

**Genetic Engineering Kills**
The messy process of genetic engineering has already taken American lives. In the late 1980s, 100 people were killed and 5,000-10,000 became sick or disabled from a disease that was named eosinophilia myalgia syndrome (EMS).[48] It started with a genetically engineered supplement, L-Tryptophan.

## Intended Consequence

The intended consequence of giving rBGH to cows is to increase milk production. Hence, it is used for economic purposes and is not intended to improve the health of the cow or the quality of the milk and meat that come from the cow.[49] Yes, some dairy cows are slaughtered for meat in the United States.[50]

Manipulating the milk supply of a cow is not a new idea. Some industrial farmers have been trying to do this for years through various methods including: selective breeding, switching from grass diets to grain-based diets, and exposing cows to long periods of artificial light. What makes rBGH unique is that it's the first genetically engineered hormone used to increase the milk supply. In fact, when the FDA approved the use of rBGH, it was the **first genetically engineered hormone** to be introduced **into our food supply**. And, it works.

rBGH reportedly increases milk production by 10-15%.[51] Therefore, in terms of its intended purpose, rBGH is an effective drug. For instance, in 1950 the typical dairy cow produced around 5,300 pounds of milk each year.[52] Today, it's common for a dairy cow to produce over 22,000 pounds of milk every year.[53] That means today's cows produce over four times more milk then they did just 60 years ago. Part of this "success" is due to genetic engineering.

On the surface, this scientific discovery sounds like a good thing. A larger milk supply means lower prices. That's great for your pocket book, but is it great for the cow? And, is rBGH great for your body?

## Unintended Consequence: Sick Cows

Over 20 medical conditions have been documented in cows treated with rBGH.[54] Some of these conditions include hoof problems that are so severe the cow can no longer walk. Other problems include: reproductive disorders, increased mastitis, digestive disorders, orthopedic problems, blood abnormalities, and a reduction in overall health including shortened life span.[54] Sadly, a 40% decrease in fertility and 55% increase in lameness have been reported in cows treated with rBGH.[55] In fact, Canada banned rBGH because it "is harmful to the health and wellness of dairy cows; it significantly increases the risk of mastitis, infertility, and lameness in cows."[51]

If rBGH-milk is the same as non-treated milk, then why is it associated with sick cows? Isn't it logical that sick cows would produce sick milk? And, couldn't sick milk be harmful to us?

## Unintended Consequence: Sick Milk

Sick cows really do produce sick milk. For instance, one of the most common side effects of rBGH injections in cows is mastitis, or inflammation of the mammary gland. rBGH-treated cows reportedly have a 33% greater chance of developing mastitis than non-treated cows.[45] The increased risk of infection may even be as high as 80%.[56] Regardless of the exact value, this is a big deal because infections, like mastitis, can lead to **pus, bacteria, and blood getting into the milk that we drink**.[54] How does that happen?

Milk is produced in the mammary gland. Common sense tells us that when a cow has an infection in the very same part of the body that produces the milk, that milk can become contaminated with pus, bacteria, and blood that were formed due to the infection. Hence, a sick cow produces sick milk.

But, don't take my word for it. Let's look at the science that supports this common-sense conclusion. Pus contains neutrophils, dead tissue cells, dead microorganisms (like bacteria) and dead white blood cells, also called somatic cells.[57] The somatic cell count is used as an indication of disease or stress in a cow. The higher the cell count, the greater the incidence of disease or stress. In other words, the somatic cell count is a scientific way of tracking infection. It also provides a way to loosely track the amount of pus in your milk. In 1994, an article published in *Nature* reported significantly more pus cells in milk from rBGH treated cows.[58] But, don't worry because the U.S. government is handling it:

**The federal government only allows roughly 178 million somatic cells per cup of milk.**[59]

That glass of milk might not look as appealing knowing that pus, including dead white blood cells and dead microorganisms, may be floating in it. But, the problem doesn't end with climbing pus cell counts.

Antibiotics are required to treat mastitis, which means **antibiotics and their byproducts are passed onto us through the milk**.[54] The use of antibiotics in cows treated with rBGH increased so dramatically that the antibiotic level in the milk climbed to levels that were not allowable by the FDA.[47] That's a problem.

There is great concern among the scientific community about the creation of superbugs. Superbugs are bacteria that we cannot readily kill with our current arsenal of antibiotics. So, if you get sick from a superbug, there may not be an antibiotic available to kill it. Superbugs are so dangerous that the Director for the CDC, Dr. Tom Frieden, called them "nightmare bacteria."[60] Superbugs are appearing largely because of our chronic exposure to antibiotics. Part of that exposure stems from our food supply. Roughly 80% of all antibiotics sold in the U.S. are fed to livestock, or farm animals. Consequently, **some of the animal products we eat are contaminated with bacteria that we cannot kill with common antibiotics.**[61]

To help counter the rise in superbugs, the FDA sets an "allowable level" of antibiotics and their residues in our milk supply. If the milk contains more antibiotic residues than the allowable level, it is thrown out. Likewise, if rBGH causes the antibiotic levels in milk to increase beyond the allowable level, rBGH should not be used in our food supply-it should be thrown out. Even the GAO expressed concern over the increase in antibiotic residues in rBGH milk. In a 1992 report, the GAO stated that the FDA should withhold approval of rBGH until the mastitis issue was resolved.[45] What did the FDA do in response to the rising level of antibiotics in milk from rBGH-treated cows?

The FDA did not stop the use of the growth hormone nor did they place a moratorium on the sale of rBGH milk until the problem was resolved. Instead, the FDA changed their regulations. They increased the allowable level of antibiotics in our milk from 1 part per 100 million to 1 part per million.[47] That's 100 times more antibiotics in our milk! Instead of addressing the culprit, rBGH, **the FDA changed its regulation to accommodate the needs of the drug.** Who did the FDA serve in this situation? Did they serve you, the consumer of the milk, or did they serve the drug company that sells rBGH?

We have one person, in particular, to thank for this change in our "food safety" policy. One individual from the FDA, Dr. Margaret Miller, changed the regulation.[47] Scientists working for the FDA were concerned about the policy change, so they wrote an anonymous letter to Congress:

"Dr. Miller [wrote] a policy on use of antimicrobials in milk. She picked an arbitrary and scientifically unsupported number…without any consumer safety testing…As you know, one big concern for BST [rBGH] is that it leads to increased antibiotic use. Monsanto [the manufacturer of rBGH] has said this is not a concern. This issue held up the approval of BST [rBGH] for a long time. Dr. Miller's policy was used as the basis for approval of BST [rBGH] despite increased antibiotic usage."[56]

Interestingly, before she was hired by the FDA, Dr. Miller worked for Monsanto where she conducted research on rBGH.[62] We will probably never know for certain if she approved rBGH because of her past connection with both Monsanto and rBGH, but the evidence is pretty damaging.

Along with more antibiotics used in rBGH-treated cows, other types of drugs are sometimes needed to treat the 19 other acknowledged illnesses that are associated with administering rBGH to cows. Like antibiotics, those drugs and their residues may bleed into the milk we drink. In addition, extra-label use drugs[‡] have reportedly been used to treat some of the illnesses caused by rBGH. For example, in a 1987 report, Monsanto revealed that cows injected with rBGH were extensively treated with drugs. Roughly 25% of those drugs were unapproved for lactating cows. In addition, no withdrawal periods were required.[54] Monsanto claims the milk from that trial was not commercialized. If it had been, it could mean that cows got sick from the rBGH treatment, they were given unapproved drugs, and their milk was collected the same day for us to drink.

But, even if the milk from that experiment wasn't commercialized, the FDA admits that illegal drug use in our dairy cows is a problem. According to the FDA, "…illegal use of veterinary drugs can be an even greater threat to the public health than the illegal use of human drugs."[63] This is a major problem because drug residues could be hazardous to us. They could ignite an immune or allergic response, or even lead to cancer if exposure is continued over time.[54]

Even worse, the FDA broke the rules when it came to testing for drug residues from rBGH. When a veterinary drug is in the experimental stage, the manufacturer of the drug is required by the FDA to create an assay to test for drug residues in the milk. That assay is supposed to be available to third parties so they can independently verify that the milk doesn't contain drug residues that might harm us. That assay exists for rBGH, but the FDA won't approve it. That means nobody is testing our milk for rBGH residues. It also means there is no verification process to determine if milk labeled as rBGH-free really is rBGH-free. So, if our milk is labeled as rBGH-free, how do we know it truly is rBGH-free?

---

‡ According to Pete Hardin, editor of *The Milkweed*, "extra-label" means veterinarians can "play God." They have "extra-label power," which allows them to use "virtually any drug in any animal" even if that drug is unapproved for use by the FDA. Those same drugs would be considered illegal if they were administered by anyone else.

According to Pete Hardin, editor of *The Milkweed*, it boils down to blindly trusting our food supply:

"In terms of the milk issue, the most egregious mistake by FDA that puts a cloud of smoke over the rest of the debate was their failure to develop a residue assay. That is the law but, in this case, they ignored it. FDA never required an assay for rBGH. Therefore, this whole debate about labeling and consumer knowledge in the dairy issue has never been properly resolved because we're going on a farmer's written certification that he's not using the drug. There have been numerous examples where that is not true. Those pledges [signed by farmers] have been violated. There is no verification in the process because FDA never required a drug residue assay for rBGH milk."[64]

So, even if your milk is labeled as rBGH-free, it may not be. That's bad news for consumers because rBGH-treated milk and non-hormone-treated milk do appear to be different. Milk from rBGH-treated cows likely has more pus, blood, antibiotic residues, and possibly residues from illegal drugs.[54] The FDA claims these two types of milk are the same, but which milk do you want to drink?

It's clear to me that sick cows really do produce sick milk. But, does sick milk lead to sick people?

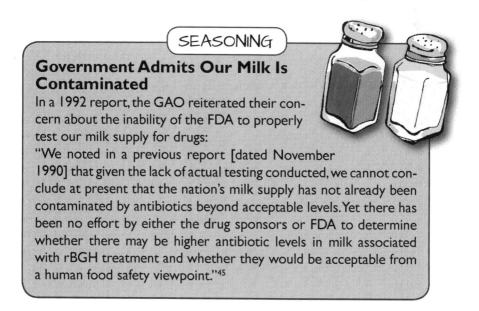

SEASONING

**Government Admits Our Milk Is Contaminated**
In a 1992 report, the GAO reiterated their concern about the inability of the FDA to properly test our milk supply for drugs:
"We noted in a previous report [dated November 1990] that given the lack of actual testing conducted, we cannot conclude at present that the nation's milk supply has not already been contaminated by antibiotics beyond acceptable levels. Yet there has been no effort by either the drug sponsors or FDA to determine whether there may be higher antibiotic levels in milk associated with rBGH treatment and whether they would be acceptable from a human food safety viewpoint."[45]

## Unintended Consequence: Sick People

As previously mentioned, there is an association between rBGH and cancer, including:

- **Colon cancer**[2–11]
- **Breast cancer**[4,12–30]
- **Childhood cancers**[31,32]
- **Prostate cancer**[33–39]

The connection between rBGH and cancer is IGF-1.

IGF-1 is a hormone that is naturally found in both cows and humans. It promotes cell growth, which is great when you need it. For example, when a cow makes milk, she needs to grow new cells. IGF-1 helps her accomplish that task. Likewise, when children and adolescents grow, IGF-1 is needed.[66] However, too much IGF-1 can be bad. Specifically, IGF-1 has been implicated in the growth of cancerous cells.[38,67,68]

That's bad news if you drink milk from rBGH-treated cows: IGF-1 has been reported in the scientific literature to be "substantially elevated" in milk from cows treated with rBGH compared with milk from untreated cows.[4,69] Additionally, the National Institute for Health reported IGF-1 levels in meat of rBGH-treated animals to be roughly twice as high as untreated animals.[70]

But, the FDA disagrees. In a document titled, "Report on the Food and Drug Administration's Review of the Safety of Recombinant Bovine Somatotropin," the FDA stated:

> "It bears repeating that the assumptions that milk levels of IGF-1 are increased following treatment with rbGH and that biologically active IGF-1 is absorbed into the body are not supported by the main body of science."[71]

Yet, in that same report, the FDA admitted that IGF-1 levels in milk were significantly increased, but the agency didn't think it was a problem:

> "Some early studies suggested that treatment of dairy cows with rbGH produced a slight, but statistically significant, increase in the average milk IGF-1 concentration. FDA determined that this modest increase in milk IGF-1 concentration was not a human food safety concern."[71]

Why does the FDA think elevated IGF-1 in milk is not a problem?

In the report, the FDA declared there is no association between IGF-1 and cancer. Yet, the agency did not provide any evidence to support the claim. But, we know from looking at the scientific literature that a connection exists. I've given you the references so you can look them up for yourself. In fact, the association between IGF-1 and cancer is so strong that Robert Cohen, author of *Milk: The Deadly Poison*, declared, "Drinking milk is the most dangerous thing we do to ourselves because it contains IGF-1." Cohen explains:

> "IGF-1 has been identified as a key factor in the growth of every human cancer. There are 4700 mammals and hundreds of millions of different proteins in nature in the animal kingdom. There is only one that is identical between two species, and it's IGF-1 in humans and cows. Not only is this the greatest coincidence in biological history, drinking milk from cows is the most dangerous thing we do to ourselves because IGF-1 is responsible for bone disease, heart disease, diabetes, and cancer. Many people will say cigarette smoking is responsible for cancer but

they cannot tell you the mechanism. I can tell you that IGF-1 promotes cancer growth-that is the mechanism."[72]

We don't have to agree that IGF-1 promotes cancer or that rBGH milk is bad for you. I encourage you to do your own homework and decide for yourself if rBGH milk is right for your family. I've provided references to get you started. The real story is *how* rBGH was approved, and the role each of us played.

## In The Dark From The Start

rBGH has been in our food supply for a long time. The FDA approved the use of the genetically engineered hormone in 1993, but we've been unknowingly drinking it since 1985.[45]

1985 was the year the FDA approved the *unrestricted* sale of milk and meat products from rBGH-treated cows. Monsanto was the manufacturer of rBGH at the time. They conducted *experiments* on cows across the United States. According to a 1992 report by the GAO, the FDA allowed Monsanto to sell the experimental milk and meat for human consumption while the drug was still in the experimental phase of development:[45]

> "We also found that food products from the rBGH-treated animals were commercially processed and sold to consumers without any labeling regarding their origin."[45]

The FDA did not require these products to be labeled.[45] **For 8 years, we drank experimental milk and ate experimental meat without even knowing it.** Clearly, the FDA didn't believe we had the right to know what we were putting in our bodies. We were un-consenting guinea pigs in a nation-wide experiment. It was funded by Monsanto and given the green light by the U.S. government, specifically the FDA. How many other foods are we unknowingly consuming that are coming from experimental drug trials?

We may never know the answer to that question because the FDA has decided it's not our right to know, and they are not obligated to tell us. According to the GAO report:

> "The FDA does not require the labeling of food products derived from animals involved in drug treatment trials…we [the GAO] believe the public should have the right to know which food

products have been produced from animals being tested with investigational drugs. Consequently, we disagree with FDA on this point."[45]

How did the FDA know that the first genetically engineered hormone was safe for us to eat while it was still undergoing testing?

It didn't. So, how could the government not tell us that we were eating experimental foods?

If you knew about rBGH, you might have chosen to drink the milk anyway. That's not the point. The FDA effectively took away our choice when they decided not to require labeling of experimental foods. It's a slow erosion of our freedom.

And, even after the FDA approved the use of rBGH in our food supply in 1993, the agency still did not tell us that our milk and meat were coming from cows that were given a genetically engineered hormone. **No labeling was required.**[45] This means that you and I had no way of knowing if our dairy products contained rBGH. They took away our choice *again*.

Where were the food companies in this nation-wide deception? Did they take the initiative and label their food products as experimental or as food that came from cows treated with genetically engineered hormones?

No.

They were complicit. Not only did they keep us in the dark, some companies tried to suppress any efforts to label dairy products. For example, some smaller farmers who were not using rBGH began labeling their milk as "hormone free." This upset Monsanto who claimed the labels were misleading. The FDA stepped in to help Monsanto, at the expense of the consumer and the small farmer, by *imposing "voluntary" labeling guidelines.* The guidelines suggested that farmers include the following statement on their label:

> "FDA states: No significant difference in milk from cows treated with artificial growth hormone."[73]

That's why the disclaimer appeared on my milk label. My milk is organic, which means it cannot come from cows treated with rBGH, since it's an artificial hormone. However, both Monsanto and our government want me to believe that rBGH-treated milk is the same as milk from cows not treated with rBGH. Hence, there is a disclaimer on the front of my milk label.

The same year the labeling guideline was released by the FDA, Monsanto began to sue small dairies for their "misleading" labels. Monsanto used the FDA's guidelines to back up their claims. For example, in 1994, Monsanto sued two small dairies, one in Texas and another in Iowa, claiming their labels were misleading because they suggested milk from rBGH-treated cows was different.[74] This was in opposition to the FDA "voluntary" guidelines. They settled out-of-court. Both dairies changed their labels as a direct result of the lawsuit.[75]

The targeting of small farms did not stop there. In 2003, Monsanto sued Oakhurst Dairy, a family-owned company, for including a statement on their label that read: "Our farmer's pledge: no artificial growth hormones."[76] They settled with Monsanto by including the FDA disclaimer on their label: "FDA states: No significant difference in milk from cows treated with artificial growth hormone."[77] So much for the labeling guidelines being "voluntary." They appear to be mandatory.

But, Monsanto took it one step further. In 2007, Monsanto petitioned the FDA and the Federal Trade Commission (FTC) to make it illegal for any company, anywhere in the U.S., to label their own products as rBGH-free. Both agencies stood up to Monsanto and denied the request. Finally, the FDA did their job! Monsanto responded by lobbying state governments. They wanted laws passed that would make it illegal for companies selling dairy products within a particular state to label their own product as rBGH-free.[78] Monsanto's efforts paid off. Ohio passed the law Monsanto desired.

Fortunately, Ohio's law was later ruled unconstitutional by the U.S. Sixth Circuit court based on the grounds that the milk from rBGH-treated cows is different than milk from cows not treated with rBGH.[79,80] According to the opinion of the judges presiding over the case (International Dairy Foods Association v Boggs), "a compositional difference does exist between milk from untreated cows and conventional milk."[80] Specifically, the court listed three reasons why rBGH milk is different than milk from cows not treated with rBGH:

1. rBGH milk contains increased levels of IGF-1.
2. There is a period of time during lactation when the milk from rBGH-treated cows has a lower nutritional quality.
3. rBGH milk contains a higher somatic cell count.

Interestingly, two government entities provided two conflicting conclusions regarding rBGH milk: One arm of the government (Sixth Circuit Court) declared rBGH milk to be different, while a second arm (the FDA) declared the milk is the same. Which government entity do you believe?

Where did the FDA come up with the disclaimer in the first place?

Michael Taylor. He was the policy director at the FDA who supervised and signed off on the disclaimer.[73] Prior to working at the FDA, he was a lawyer for King & Spaulding. Monsanto was one of their clients.[62]

## Let's recap:

- We were un-consenting guinea pigs for 8 years (1985-1993).
- Evidence suggests that rBGH milk contains elevated levels of IGF-1, which is associated with various cancers and premature development in children.
- Most industrialized countries won't import our milk.
- The Sixth Circuit court disagrees with the FDA, stating that rBGH milk is different from non-rBGH milk.
- Yet, to this day, the FDA tells us that rBGH milk is safe for us to consume and is the same as milk from non-hormone treated cows. Consequently, they still do not require our dairy products to be labeled.

Does something seem off to you?

Our rBGH story looks pretty bad for the FDA right now. But, before we jump to any conclusions, let's figure out the FDA's side of the story. Maybe I'm being overly optimistic, but I need to believe that the FDA did not knowingly put us at risk. Why would they tell us the milk is not harmful if it might actually hurt us? That just doesn't make sense. What would they have to gain by lying to us? I need to believe the FDA based their decision on sound, solid science and not on pressure from industry and their lobbyists. I need to believe the FDA is protecting the American people. After all, we pay them to watch over our food supply. So, why would they knowingly make us sick? We need to go directly to the source.

## FDA Review Of rBGH

In a 1999 report, the FDA revealed that the **first genetically engineered hormone was released into our food supply based primarily on two rat studies**. They didn't even conduct the studies themselves! Monsanto conducted both studies. And, we're not allowed to see the data. The FDA won't release it. Instead, the agency refers to an article published in *Science* in 1990 to back up their claim that milk from rBGH-treated cows is safe for humans.

That article in *Science* was used to green light the drug. Unfortunately, the authors of that study were not independent scientists. At the time the article was published, one of the authors worked at the FDA Center for Veterinary Medicine, Office of New Animal Drug Evaluation in Maryland. The second author was a former employee with the same office of the FDA.[81]

In addition, the article was published *three years before* the FDA approved rBGH. Wrap your mind around that one: The FDA publically championed the safety of rBGH three years before the review of the drug had been completed.[81]

In the *Science* article, the two rat studies were briefly discussed. According to the FDA scientists, "Negative results were obtained with oral administration of rbGH in all studies."[81] However, the studies are listed as "unpublished reports," which means we can't look at the data for ourselves.[81] Instead, we have to take the word of the drug companies and the FDA scientists at face value.

The FDA scientists claimed that the studies showed no changes in organ weights or tissues, indicating that rBGH did not have an effect on the rats.[81] This claim is critical. If there were changes in organ weights, it would warrant long-term safety studies. But, because there were no reported changes, long-term safety studies were not required. But, was the data accurate?

The limited data provided in the *Science* article tells a different story. According to Dr. Samuel Epstein, the organ weights did change:

> "FDA fraudulently misrepresented Monsanto's claims that the weight of organs of rats dosed orally with rBGH or IGF-1 were unchanged, rather than in fact increased, by presenting the data in absolute values rather than relative to whole body weights."[54]

Additionally, as reported by Jeffrey Smith, founder of the Institute for Responsible Technology, "while the authors indicated that the weights of many organs and tissues were measured at the end of the ninety-day feeding study, the *Science* article listed the data for only four of them."[47]

What happened to the rest of the data?

Robert Cohen, author of *Milk: The Deadly Poison*, tried to track down the organ data. When Mr. Cohen asked the FDA in 1994 for the rest of the organ weights, he was told the measurements were a "trade secret."[47] This was baffling because in 1992, the Inspector General of the Department of Health and Human Services, Richard P. Kusserow, stated that "complete disclosure of bst data will not occur unless and until FDA approves the drug for commercial use."[70] At the time of Mr. Cohen's request, rBGH had already been approved, so why was the data not released to the public?

After reaching a dead-end with the FDA, Mr. Cohen reached out to Monsanto. He was refused. Next, he filed a Freedom of Information Act request for the study. That was also refused. He tried the FDA again, and was refused again. The FDA said, "Release of information would cause substantial competitive and financial harm to the company [Monsanto]."[56] Then, Mr. Cohen sued in Federal Court, but the Court ruled against him saying that the organ weights were a trade secret and if people knew what they were it could lead to "competitive and substantial harm" to Monsanto.[56] Why the secrecy? If the organ weights truly didn't change then why not show us the data?

If you recall, the FDA would not admit, in their safety report, that IGF-1 levels in rBGH milk were elevated. Well, the FDA scientists who wrote the *Science* article admitted that IGF-1 is elevated. According to the article:

> "Recombinant bGH treatment produces an increase in the concentration of insulin-like growth factor-I (IGF-I) in cow's milk."[82]

However, the FDA scientists claimed that IGF-1 is not orally active because organ weights did not change. Again, we cannot confirm this conclusion without knowing the organ weights.

The FDA scientists also claimed that milk from rBGH-treated cows was safe for humans because even if the milk contained elevated levels of bGH (a 26% increase was reported in the article), it is destroyed when milk is pasteurized. According to the FDA scientists:

> "It has also been determined that at least 90% of bGH activity is destroyed upon pasteurization of milk.[47] Therefore, bGH residues do not present a human food safety concern."[81]

This claim is backed by a study conducted by Paul Groenewegen, who was an undergraduate at the time.[81] Three of his co-authors had close ties to Monsanto. They either conducted research for Monsanto or had previously published with Monsanto scientists.[48,56] Their study contains a fatal flaw: They heated "the milk to 69°C [156.2°F] – 71°C [159.8°F] for 25-30 min."[83] If they were trying to mimic the U.S. standard pasteurization protocol, heating the milk to roughly 156-160°F would require heat treatment for roughly 15 seconds. Certainly, the milk would not be heated for 25-30 minutes at that high of a temperature. In other words, they pasteurized the milk 120 times longer than normal, as reported by Robert Cohen.[56] In a testimony before an FDA panel, Robert Cohen claimed, "They [the scientists] intentionally tried to destroy the hormone."[84]

But, the pasteurization process they followed didn't even work! As Cohen explains, it only destroyed "19 percent of the BST in milk from cows treated with BST."[56] After that didn't work:

> "[T]hey added 146 times the level of naturally occurring bST in powdered form to the milk and heated it. The powdered rbST in milk was destroyed! They saved the day for Monsanto…These men of science could claim that heat treatment destroys bST."[56]

In Cohen's testimony before the FDA panel, he explained what happened next:

> "And at that moment, FDA said to Monsanto, 'Because you destroy it by pasteurization, you don't have to do further toxicology studies. You don't have to develop a test for this hormone in milk. It's now safe to drink.' They [FDA] developed a zero day withdrawal—they determined it was safe to drink."[84]

In the end, the FDA declared milk from rBGH-treated cows to be safe based, in part, on unpublished industry data, partially disclosed organ weights, and a pasteurization study where the milk was cooked 120 times longer than normal and then "spiked" with powdered hormone.[56] Based on that limited information, the FDA declared no long-term studies were required:

> "...long-term toxicity studies to ascertain human health safety were not required by FDA or conducted by Monsanto."[71]

This statement is at the heart of the rBGH debate. This one sentence sparked an onslaught of criticism and outrage from consumers, scientists, and reputable organizations. Arguably, the entire debate over the potential harmful effects of rBGH hinges on that one statement. How do we know this genetically engineered hormone is not harmful to cows, humans, or the environment, if there are no long-term studies?

We simply cannot know. Once the FDA decided not to require long-term safety studies of rBGH, and instead approved the use of the first genetically engineered hormone in our milk based on unpublished industry data, it opened itself up to an unending barrage of criticism that has persisted for over 20 years.

As I poured over the available data, I kept coming back to the same question: Why would the FDA approve the first genetically engineered hormone in our food supply based largely on two industry-funded, short-term studies on rats?

I couldn't find an adequate answer to that question. Then, I realized I was asking the wrong question. The more important question is: *Why* did rBGH get approved? Who stood to gain from the FDA approving rBGH?

The manufacturer of rBGH: Monsanto.

## Taken At Face Value

Health Canada, the Canadian version of our FDA, conducted an audit of the rBGH approval process. They discovered that the rats in one of the short-term studies showed "a distinct immunological effect" from consuming rBGH. That finding means that long-term studies should have been conducted. Health Canada concluded that the rBGH "evaluation was largely a theoretical review taking the manufacturer's conclusions at face value."[49] In other words, Monsanto said the drug was safe and the FDA believed them even though the evidence did not support that claim.

## The Machine

Monsanto stood to make millions of dollars each year from selling rBGH. Thus, it was in their best interest to get rBGH approved and accepted by the public. How did they do it? How did Monsanto get the most powerful country in the world to approve the first genetically modified food even though it made cows sick, likely contributes to cancer growth, and was banned by most other industrialized countries?

They succeeded by creating what I like to call The Machine. There are 7 major parts that make up The Machine. Let's begin with the revolving door.

### 1. Revolving Door

We've already encountered the revolving door twice in our rBGH story. If you recall, Michael Taylor pushed through the FDA "voluntary" milk labeling guidelines. Even though the FDA claims these milk-labeling guidelines were "voluntary," they were used by Monsanto to sue dairy farmers who tried to label their milk as "rBGH free." Mr. Taylor moved back and forth between the FDA and Monsanto. He was an attorney for the company that represented Monsanto, and then became Vice President of Monsanto. Later, he was appointed by President Bush to be the FDA Deputy Commissioner of Policy (1991-1994). That's when he wrote the FDA's labeling guidelines for rBGH. Then, Mr. Taylor went back to work for Monsanto. Later, President Obama reappointed him to the FDA as the Food Safety Czar.[41]

Dr. Margaret Miller was another key player in the approval of rBGH. She was responsible for increasing the allowable level of antibiotic residue in milk. Dr. Miller worked for Monsanto from 1985-1989 as a Laboratory Supervisor, where she worked on bovine growth hormone. Then, in 1989, President George H.W. Bush appointed her to the FDA. She was the FDA Branch Chief of Hormones, Pharmacological Agents. That division of the FDA evaluated the same research on rBGH that Dr. Miller conducted while working for Monsanto.[62]

But, the connections between Monsanto and government run much deeper than Mr. Taylor and Dr. Miller. An investigation by the GAO revealed that the FDA's primary reviewer of rBGH was Dr. Susan Sechen. She helped rBGH gain FDA approval by reviewing and approving her own studies! She conducted studies on Monsanto's rBGH drug as a graduate student at Cornell and then she was hired by the FDA to review those very same studies.[62] Additionally, Dr. Sechen was "publishing articles in support of Monsanto and rBGH while still an FDA employee," according to Dr. Samuel Epstein, author of *What's In Your Milk?*[54]

Another connection between government and industry is Dr. Michael Friedman. He was the Deputy Commissioner of the FDA before becoming the Chief Clinical Researcher of Monsanto's G.D. Searle unit.[54]

Sadly, the close ties between Monsanto and government don't stop with the FDA. It also extends to the EPA, Congress, and even the White House:

- Ann Veneman was on the Board of Directors of a Monsanto Subsidiary and in 2001 she was appointed by President George W. Bush to be the U.S. Secretary of Agriculture.[85]
- Supreme Court Justice Clarence Thomas worked as an attorney for Monsanto.[86]
- Roger Beachy was the Director at Danforth Center for Monsanto. In 2009, he was appointed by President Obama to be the Director of the USDA National Institute of Food and Agriculture.[87]
- Former Secretary of Health, Tommy Thompson, received $50,000 from biotech companies during his election campaign for governor of Wisconsin. After elected, he declared Wisconsin

to be a "biotech zone" so that Monsanto could use rBGH in that state even though dairy farmers opposed the plan.[85]

- Representative Richard Pombo (R-CA) led the Agriculture Sub-committee on Dairy, Livestock and Poultry. He helped stall the 1994 bill that would have made labeling milk containing rBGH mandatory. The bill was killed in committee. Pombo took campaign money from Monsanto.[85]
- The former U.S. Trade Ambassador, Mickey Cantor, ended up on Monsanto's board.[54]
- Former Secretary of Agriculture and Iowa governor, Thomas Vilsack, established and chaired the Governors Biotechnology Partnership group. The Biotechnology Industry Organization named him "Governor of the Year" in 2001. Monsanto is a member of that organization. Then, in 2009, he was appointed as the U.S. Secretary of Agriculture under Obama. He is reportedly an advocate of genetically modified foods.[87]
- William Ruckelshaws moved from the EPA to Monsanto.[54]
- Linda Fisher moved from the EPA to Monsanto. President Clinton appointed her in 2001 as the EPA Deputy Administrator. Later, she became the Vice President of Government and Public Affairs for Monsanto.[54]
- Marcia Hale moved from the White House to Monsanto.[54]
- Jack Watson was Chief of Staff for President Jimmy Carter before he was hired as a lawyer for Monsanto.[54]

## 2. Manipulation and Suppression

A handful of FDA employees came forward to inform the public about what happened behind the scenes at the FDA. One of these brave men is Dr. Richard Burroughs, who worked for the FDA for 10 years. During that time, he oversaw the rBGH field trial.[88] According to Dr. Burroughs:

> "[FDA] decided to cover up inappropriate studies and decisions...[They] suppressed and manipulated data to cover up their own ignorance and incompetence."[89]

Alexander Apostolou, former Director of the FDA's Division of Toxicology, also came forward with claims regarding inappropriate agency behavior. In an affidavit, he revealed the following:

"Sound scientific procedures for evaluating human food safety of veterinary drugs have been disregarded. I have faced continuous pressure from my CVM [Center for Veterinary Medicine] superiors to reach scientific conclusions favorable to the drug industry...In my time at CVM I have witnessed drug manufacturer sponsors improperly influence the agency's scientific analysis, decision-making, and fundamental mission." He also stated that the agency's pattern is keeping "industry content through uncritical acceptance of sponsor's claims and data, and...bending the rules to make their data look acceptable."[89]

But, the most damaging evidence of data manipulation and suppression comes from files that were allegedly stolen from the FDA and sent to Dr. Samuel Epstein, the head of the Cancer Prevention Coalition. He published the documents in *The Milkweed* in 1990.[88] Those confidential files contained the data that was submitted by Monsanto to the FDA for approval of rBGH. The information was telling.

Remember how FDA scientists claimed, in the *Science* article, that the organ weights from the rat studies did not change? And, when Robert Cohen tried to gain access to the data he was denied because they are considered a trade secret? The confidential company files reveal that cows receiving rBGH had enlarged organs including: ovaries, hearts, livers, kidneys, and adrenal glands.[88] In fact, "ovary sizes in treated cows were ostensibly larger than ovaries in control cows."[88] The Milkweed reported that the abnormalities were "dismissed by Monsanto as 'harmless physiological shifts'."[88]

The confidential company files also confirm reproductive problems among rBGH-treated cows. For example, rBGH-treated cows had a significant drop in pregnancy rate:

> "95% of control cows open at the start of the trial became pregnant. 52% of bGH-treated cows open at the start of the trial became pregnant."[88]

In addition,[§] illegal drug use was exposed in the confidential company files. According to *The Milkweed*:

---

§ Pete Hardin acknowledges that the use of the work "illegal" is appropriate because veterinarians have "extra-label power" allowing them to give virtually any drug to any animal. These drugs are considered "illegal" unless a veterinarian administers them.

"Illegal drug use by Monsanto employees on bGH [rBGH] test cows is documented for FDA, in Monsanto's NADA files. Drugs used to illegally treat milking cows at Monsanto's research farm include: Banamine, Di-Trim, Gentamycin, Ivomec, Oxytet, Piperallin, Rompun and Vetislud…one cow…received over 120 drug treatments in a single lactation. Nearly half of those treatments were with illegal drugs."[88]

One of those drugs, Rompun, is only supposed to be used in horses, according to the FDA. Additionally, the drug label for Rompun states, "the drug may not be injected into horses to be slaughtered for food."[90] That's a problem for us because the "FDA sets no milk and meat withdrawal times for non-approved drugs."[90] Do you recall that Monsanto claimed the milk from their experimental trial was not sold for our consumption? According to *The Milkweed*, Monsanto's "records do not indicate whether milk from Monsanto research cows treated with illegal drugs was withheld from the market."[88] Consequently, you and I may have drunk milk containing illegal drugs. We may still be drinking illegal drugs in our milk today.

In addition, Monsanto's own files reveal there was "up to a 1200-fold increase in blood levels" of bGH following drug treatment during Monsanto's experiment.[90] When a hormone increases in the blood 1200 times, it's logical to expect some of that hormone will end up in the milk. How much hormone do you think ends up in the milk when blood levels skyrocket 1200-fold?

As we previously learned, the hormone we are most concerned with is IGF-1. And, based on the article published in *Science* by FDA employees, we know IGF-1 is elevated in milk from rBGH-treated cows:

"Recombinant bGH treatment produces an increase in the concentration of insulin-like growth factor-I (IGF-I) in cow's milk."[82]

I wonder how much IGF-1 ends up in milk when BGH blood levels increase 1200 times? Regardless, the stolen files reveal that milk from cows treated with rBGH is different, and the FDA acknowledged that difference.

Internal FDA correspondence contained within the confidential company files reveal that the elevated blood levels of BGH "prompted FDA to institute withdrawal time for meat and milk of bGH-treated cows, when trials started in the early 1980s. Until 1985 or so, FDA required a five-day withdrawal period following the last injection for treated dairy cows. Meat from treated cows could not be slaughtered for 15 days following the final bGH shots."[90] In other words, early on in the rBGH drug trials, the FDA did its job. They acknowledged that elevated blood hormone levels could lead to elevated milk and meat levels. Consequently, they required withdrawal periods.

So, what happened? Why were the mandatory withdrawal periods removed in 1985?

Monsanto wanted the withdrawal periods removed, so they conducted a 28-day feeding study on rats. A memorandum from the Department of Heath & Human Services, dated February 20, 1987, was published in *The Milkweed* that confirms the removal of the withdrawal period based on a single rat study:

> "The firm [Monsanto] submitted a 28-day oral feeding study in rats that demonstrated no oral activity…based on the results of this study, the sponsor was granted a zero withdrawal and milk discard period for cows treated with daily injections of up to 40 mg/head/day. The sponsor was also granted a zero withdrawal and milk discard period for lactating dairy cattle treated with a sustained-release formulation containing 750 mg of [rBGH] injected at 14-day intervals…Based on the results of the oral feeding study and our knowledge of the characteristics and biological activity of bovine somatotropin, we have no objection to granting the sponsor's requests."[90]

When the FDA removed the withdrawal period for milk and meat coming from rBGH-treated cows, it didn't just remove that restriction from Monsanto. The FDA removed the withdrawal period for all manufacturers of rBGH. According to *The Milkweed*:

> "Monsanto's one-time, 28-day rat feeding trial became the basis for allowing all bGH trial milk and meat to be consumed by humans with no withdrawal period."[90]

Based on the culmination of the evidence revealed in the confidential industry files, Dr. Esptein and Peter Hardin, *The Milkweed* editor, accused the FDA and Monsanto of suppressing and misrepresenting scientific data:

"Monsanto's latest admission of the very high blood bGH levels, coupled with their own data…on elevated bGH milk levels, fully supports our position that both industry and the FDA have suppressed and grossly misrepresented information on elevated bGH levels in blood and milk, both are critical public health concerns."[90]

*Let's Recap:*

- FDA employees revealed that data suppression and manipulation occurred.
- Confidential industry files revealed:
  o The use of "illegal" drugs.
  o A dramatic increase in growth hormone levels in blood (coupled with an admission of elevated levels of hormone in rBGH milk)
  o Enlarged organs in cows treated with rBGH.
  o Decreased fertility in cows treated with rBGH.
  o No required withdrawal period before selling the milk for our consumption.

## SEASONING

### Harsh Words From Congress

In May of 1990, after reading the leaked confidential files, Congressman John Conyers wrote a letter to the Inspector General stating:

"I find it reprehensible that Monsanto and the FDA have chosen to suppress and manipulate animal health test data."[91]

In addition, Congressman Conyers expressed concern about the lack of available research on human safety, the potential for high levels of rBGH in milk (based on the industry files), and the withholding of critical research pertaining to the safety of rBGH from the public.[91] Unfortunately, his inquiry went nowhere.

## 3. Intimidation and Retribution

On October 22, 1998, three scientists from Health Canada, the Canadian version of the FDA, testified against rBGH approval in front of a Canadian Senate Commission. One of the whistleblowers was Dr. Shiv Chopra. He worked for Health Canada for roughly 36 years. Dr. Chopra claimed that he and other scientists at Health Canada were pressured by both Senior Canadian officials and Monsanto to approve rBGH:

> "We have been pressured and coerced to pass drugs of questionable safety, including rBST [rBGH]."[92]

At the Senate hearing, Dr. Chopra revealed that every file related to rBGH was "now controlled by one senior bureaucrat and can only be viewed by gaining permission."[92] He also told the Senate committee that the job of scientists at Health Canada was to "serve the client" and that the "client is now the industry" instead of the people of Canada. A second scientist testified that:

> "Pharmaceutical manufacturers have far too much influence in the drug approval process. [Scientists] often feel that their careers are threatened if they stand in the way of a drug they don't believe is safe. [And] managers without scientific experience regularly overrule their decisions."[93]

At the hearing, the three scientists were asked if anyone from Monsanto had lobbied them. Margaret Haydon, DVM (Health Canada, 1983-2004) replied, "I did attend a meeting back approximately in 1989, 1990, and Monsanto representatives had met with myself and my supervisor...and at that meeting an offer of $1 to $2 million was made by the company..."[48] According to Dr. Chopra, "Monsanto did not deny that they made the offer of $1 to $2 million at this meeting. They later on tried to say, 'oh this was an offer of research in Canada to do some more studies.' That's what happened in Canada."[48]

After the hearing, Dr. Chopra admitted that he was intimidated:

> "My question to myself was, 'What truth am I going to tell? The one I know or the one the ministry is telling me to tell?'... Ultimately the buck stops at the scientist evaluating. That's me. And, if I agree then I'm part of the corruption. If I don't agree, I get fired. I chose to be fired."[48]

Dr. Chopra chose to stand on principle. He told the truth and it paid off for the citizens of Canada. The testimony of those brave scientists helped ban rBGH in Canada. It was a victory for Canadian citizens. Sadly, those 3 brave individuals would pay a steep price for their honesty. According to Dr. Chopra:

> "The European Parliament, based on the revelations in Canada, banned it [rBGH] forever. And, then all of a sudden we three [the three whistleblowers] were dismissed for disobedience. All three of us were fired and those fights are now in court."[48]

The lesson learned from the Canadian situation was: You stand against The Machine, you get crushed.

Intimidation also ran deep here in the United States. For instance, FDA employees sent an anonymous letter to Congress in 1994. They were intimidated and were afraid of retribution from a government employee with close ties to industry:

> "We are afraid to speak openly about the situation because of retribution from our director, Dr. Robert Livingston. Dr. Livingston openly harasses anyone who states an opinion in opposition to his…This is not the first time that CVM [Center for Veterinary Medicine] employees have charged Dr. Livingston with fraud and abuse leading to endangerment of the public safety. However, it seems if anyone speaks out, they, not Dr. Livingston, end up in trouble. We, as government employees, cannot understand why it is allowed to continue."[56]

In addition, a few FDA employees challenged the approval of rBGH. One of those heroes was the veterinarian in charge of the review of rBGH, Dr. Richard Burroughs. According to Dr. Burroughs, FDA officials "suppressed and manipulated data" in order to approve the drug application.[89] Additionally, Dr. Burroughs said the submitted data was insufficient:

> "The data they [Monsanto] came in with lacked a lot of insight into the dairy industry. They didn't ask crucial questions about diseases like mastitis, which is infection of the mammary gland, and reproductive problems. So when the first data came in and that was missing I said, 'Alright guys, you need to go back and get information.' So that set it back probably two or three years."[48]

HANDS OFF MY FOOD!

Monsanto also only looked at one milk cycle. Consequently, Dr. Burroughs couldn't determine if the hormone affected newborn calves or subsequent periods of lactation. Then, he requested toxicology and immunology tests.[47] **A month later he was fired for alleged incompetence.** He had worked as a veterinarian for the FDA for roughly 10 years. As reported by Jeffrey Smith, Dr. Burroughs recalled, "I was told that I was slowing down the approval process."[94] He continues, "They [the FDA] pretty much just sidetracked me. My boss pulled in other people that were closer to him and I saw less and less of the data. Eventually, I was fired. I was escorted to the door and told that was it. I was done."[48]

Dr. Burroughs later revealed his opinion of the FDA review process:

"There seemed to be a trend in place toward approval at any price. It went from a university-like setting where there was independent scientific review to an atmosphere of 'approve, approve, approve'…the thinking [at the FDA] is, 'How many things can we approve this year?' Somewhere along the way they abdicated their responsibility to the public welfare."[89]

He also expressed his concern with the approval of rBGH. According to Dr. Burroughs:

"Well, the whole rBGH thing represents fundamental flaws in the regulatory process. The outside influence, the lack of proper structure, proper personnel to do the job that we trust them to do. The FDA does no studies. The companies do the studies and send the paperwork to the FDA who then reviews it…I found flaws in it that, according to regulation, good science should have been addressed. This was approved prematurely without adequate information."[95]

His story doesn't end there. According to Dr. Burroughs, he was threatened "…mainly by the lawyers for Monsanto because when I was going for my appeal they told my lawyer that if I went in and revealed any company secrets in my defense they would sue me." The FDA was forced to reinstate him. However, Dr. Burroughs later resigned.[48]

Why was a veterinarian in charge of reviewing the drug submission anyway? The drug was given to cows, but humans consumed the milk and meat. Thus, shouldn't an expert in human health and human medicine have reviewed the drug?

**The FDA utilized a short cut in the review process by viewing rBGH as an animal drug and not a human drug. That distinction allowed them to avoid the more extensive and time-consuming approval process that is required for human drugs.** "A human drug requires two years of carcinogenicity tests and birth defect testing," according to William von Meyer, PhD a Research Scientists at the FDA.[48] In other words, rBGH should have been extensively tested for 2 years. Instead, according to Dr. Meyer, "BGH [rBGH] was tested 90 days on 30 rats…before it was approved."[48]

The intimidation and retribution Dr. Burroughs received was not an isolated incidence at the FDA. Joseph Settepani was an FDA chemist in charge of quality control for veterinary drugs. At a public hearing held by a New York congressman, Mr. Settepani stated there was:

"…a systematic human food safety breakdown at the Center for Veterinary Medicine."[89]

Shortly after, he was "reprimanded for insubordination, threatened with dismissal, and stripped of his duties as a supervisor." Later, at a hearing in front of a congressional subcommittee, Settepani revealed that he was sent to work at a trailer located on an experimental farm. He was removed from any policy-making decisions regarding human food safety. Settepani told the subcommittee that "dissent is not tolerated if it could seriously threaten industry profits."[89]

Intimidation wasn't restricted to government employees. The Machine reached independent scientists who spoke out against rBGH as well. One such victim was Dr. David Kronfeld. Dr. Kronfeld was a leading researcher in bovine growth hormone. In the 1960s, he warned that bovine growth hormone residues might have negative health effects on humans and he advocated for more research to be conducted. Consequently, he was "frozen out" of research money that would have allowed him to study bovine growth hormone.[88] He was vindicated when a manufacturer of rBGH, Elanco, admitted in their drug application that the bovine growth hormone fragments were active in humans:

"Tryptic digests of bGH produce some metabolic effects in hypopituitary humans similar to those effects noted after administration of HGH (human growth hormone)."[54,96]

Those tryptic digests might have been one reason why a withdrawal period was required in the 1980s.[54] We know that a letter was sent from the FDA to Monsanto in 1982 acknowledging that rBGH-treated cows had higher blood hormone levels and, therefore, withdrawal periods were recommended:

> "Based on these data...FDA recommends that a milk-discard period of 5 days and a withdrawal period of 15 days prior to slaughter be observed..."[54]

It's interesting to note that Dr. Kronfeld was practically ostracized from the growth hormone scientific community for recommending that growth hormone fragments be studied in more detail. Yet, the FDA likely set a withdrawal period for milk and meat consumed from rBGH-treated cows based on the same concern. Of even greater concern is what happened next. According to *The Milkweed*:

> "In recent years, Kronfeld's letters and articles in veterinary journals have raised doubt about the design of animal health tests. Kronfeld has criticized manipulation of animal health data from field trials on reproduction and mastitis. For his 'heresy,' a Monsanto employee (Dr. Winston Samuel of Liverpool, NY) wrote three letters to VPI [Virginia Polytechnic Institute] during 1989 implicitly threatening that Monsanto might cease all research grants to that university if Kronfeld didn't silence his criticism of bGH research. Academic freedom?"[88]

*Let's recap:*

- Whistleblowers at Health Canada helped ban rBGH in Canada and were later fired.
- Principled FDA employees and independent scientists who dared to question rBGH were intimidated and sometimes fired.

## 4. Indentured Scientists

The FDA does not conduct studies on food safety. Instead, the agency relies on industry to demonstrate the safety of their products. The FDA does, however, inspect clinical experiments when the research is part of

FDA human drug trials. Unfortunately, the FDA doesn't actively tell the public about its findings. Consequently, the *Journal of the American Medical Association of Internal Medicine* (*JAMA*), a renowned medical journal, published a study detailing the findings of the FDA inspections between 1998 and 2013. They analyzed FDA documents that cited evidence of "objectionable conditions or practices." *JAMA* only reported on studies that had been published in the scientific literature. What they found is shocking.

According to *JAMA*, **39% of the clinical trials contained falsified data**.[97] Furthermore, the FDA largely ignored these violations:

> "When the FDA finds significant departures from good clinical practice, those findings are seldom reflected in the peer-reviewed literature, even when there is evidence of data fabrication or other forms of research misconduct."[97]

Why are so many scientists falsifying data?

The pressure within the scientific world is immense. Funding is critical for survival in academia. If you lose your grant money, you might as well pack up your desk and escort yourself out through the back door of the university. That's why these scientists are often referred to as indentured scientists.[54] To receive funding, you must publish your research findings in reputable scientific journals. Whoever controls what gets published, controls the scientific world. So, who is controlling the publications?

Five corporate publishing groups control more than half of the market for scientific journal articles, according to researchers from the University of Montreal.[98] They analyzed all of the scientific literature between 1973 and 2013 and found that large companies have gobbled up smaller publishers. That's a problem because the large companies often favor large industries like drug and vaccine companies, including Monsanto. In addition, "academic research groups have become increasingly beholden to the interests of these major publishers." As a consequence, scientists are less independent and published studies are more biased towards what's best for industry. According to *Natural News*,

> "The result is a publishing oligopoly in which scientists are muzzled by an overarching trend toward politically correct, and industry-favoring, 'science.'"[99]

This is a difficult situation to correct because, as previously mentioned, indentured scientists rely on grant money to keep their jobs. To get grant money, you have to get published. You are more likely to get published if your study findings are in alignment with the agenda of your publisher. According to the lead author from the Montreal study:

> "As long as publishing in high impact factor journals is a requirement for researchers to obtain positions, research funding, and recognition from peers, the major commercial publishers will maintain their hold on the academic publishing system."[99]

## Let's recap:

- The scientific publishing world is controlled by a handful of companies that tend to favor industry.
- Therefore, some scientists falsify data to ensure their own professional survival.
- Consequently, the public will continue to be bombarded with conflicting evidence on every scientific issue imaginable, including what's "good" and what's "bad" to eat.

## 5. Silencing the Media

Monsanto's PR firm helped create the Dairy Coalition in 1989.[100] The Dairy Coalition had an enormous amount of influence in determining which foods made it into our food supply, including products from rBGH-treated cows. The coalition members included the following:

- American Farm Bureau Federation: This is the group that later lobbied for "food disparagement laws." Oprah Winfrey was sued under that law in Texas.[101]
- International Food Information Council: They are funded by industry. When safety and health concerns arise about food, this group publicly discredits the opposition.[54]
- Grocery Manufacturers of America: They pick which foods are on our grocery store shelves.
- Food Marketing Institute: An advocate for industry.
- American Dietetic Association (Now called the Academy of Nutrition and Dietetics): It's the largest group of food and

nutrition professionals in the world. It includes dietitians and nutritionists in all areas of life, such as hospitals, schools, long-term care facilities, businesses, and home health care. This group advises us on what to eat. They receive money from industry.

- Academic consultants: These are the "experts" we previously discussed that are often bought and paid for by industry.
- National Association of State Departments of Agriculture: This group represents the top dogs in the Departments of Agriculture in all 50 states.

One of the ways the Dairy Coalition exerted its influence is by controlling brand messaging. For instance, in the late 1980s, a public relations firm was hired to rank reporters as friends or enemies. If a reporter made the enemy list, the Dairy Coalition would pressure their editors. **Consequently, the media was largely complicit in the deception of the public.**[54]

Additionally, Monsanto threatened media networks and individual reporters who tried to tell the rBGH story. In fact, two reporters from the Tampa Bay FOX station were fired when they refused to stop reporting on the issue.[54]

Jane Akre and Steve Wilson were investigating rBGH. They interviewed farmers who witnessed health problems in their cows after treating them with rBGH. Akre and Wilson also interviewed Monsanto scientists and Canadian government officials who claimed Monsanto tried to bribe them. In addition, they interviewed Dr. Epstein, who provided scientific evidence supporting the association between rBGH and various cancers, specifically through increased IGF-1.[54]

The report was scheduled to air on February 24, 1997. By that time, the station Akre and Wilson worked for had been sold to Rupert Murdoch's Fox network. Shortly before the report aired, Monsanto's attorneys contacted the Fox network. According to Dr. Epstein, the lawyers were "charging that Akre and Wilson had blatantly assaulted 'their integrity and the integrity of their product POSILAC (rBGH).'"[54] Additionally, "Monsanto denied that IGF-1 levels were increased in rBGH milk, that such increased levels posed cancer risks and that IGF-1 causes malignant transformation of normal human cells." Fox offered Monsanto an additional interview where they could "correct any misinformation." According to Dr. Epstein, "Monsanto immediately replied with a still more threatening letter." Fox backed down. Akre and Wilson were allowed to air their report, but the content had to be "mandated scripts."[54]

Akre and Wilson objected to the mandated script. They tried to work with Fox. They rewrote the script many times over a nine-month period. Fox refused any rewrites unless the script contained all of the mandated changes. When, Akre and Wilson refused, Fox offered a cash settlement with a gag order attached. Akre and Wilson refused the offer and were fired on December 2, 1997.[54]

Akre and Wilson sued "for declaratory relief and damages." The attorneys for Fox unsuccessfully tried to bar Dr. Epstein's testimony. In August of 2000, a jury decided against Fox, stating they violated the whistleblower law. Akre was awarded $425,000 in damages. The jury found that, "Akre suffered unlawful retaliation by Fox after she threatened to disclose to the Federal Communications Commission the 'broadcast of a false, distorted, or slanted news report.'" However, Fox won on appeal. Fox attorneys argued:

> "...technically there was no violation of state whistleblower laws because technically it is not against any law, rule or regulation to lie to the public over the public airways."[54]

Where do the news organizations draw the line when it comes to lying to the public? Can we trust the news to provide accurate reports?

Akre and Wilson stood up for the truth and were crushed by The Machine. Not only was the network's behavior accepted by our legal system, it was rewarded. Akre and Wilson ended up having to pay Fox "a low six-figure sum" for appellate costs. That was substantially lower than the $2 million Fox wanted them to pay as a "reasonable reimbursement."[54]

## 6. Medical Associations

The Machine also infiltrated medical associations, including the American Cancer Society (ACS) and the American Dietetic Association (ADA). Both are mainstream institutions and medical authorities in the United States. They are *trusted* scientific organizations. When they make recommendations, people listen, which is scary because they both took cues from Monsanto's Machine.

For instance, the Dairy Coalition has advised these medical associations on how to respond to inquiries from the press about the safety of dairy products, including milk. On September 21, 1995, the Cancer Prevention Coalition, headed by Dr. Epstein, held a press conference to unveil the "dirty dozen." It was a list of foods containing carcinogens and other potentially harmful chemicals. That year, milk earned the #2 spot among the worst offenders. Hot dogs took the top spot.

The Dairy Coalition found out about the press conference and quickly mobilized The Machine. According to a Dairy Coalition memorandum dated September 22, 1995, the Dairy Coalition prepared talking points for the American Cancer Society before they spoke with the media:

> "We [the Dairy Coalition] kept in close contact with the American Cancer Society, whose experts have already been briefed on bST [rBGH]/milk safety issues, to help them prepare for questions from reporters, the…information we gave them was distributed to their offices around the country."[54]

Not surprisingly, the talking point from the American Cancer Society was the following: "The evidence for potential harm [of rBGH] to humans is inconclusive. More research is needed to help better address these concerns."[102] The memorandum also revealed a close relationship between the Dairy Coalition and the American Dietetic Association:

> "We advised the Washington, D.C. 'Ambassador' from the American Dietetic Association, who often attends such events and provides commentary and nutritional information to the news media."[54]

Keep in mind that the American Dietetic Association is the group of "experts" who, according to their website, "play a key role in shaping the public's food choices." They also provide "expert testimony at hearings" and lobby Congress regarding federal and state food regulations.[103] It's pretty scary to realize that Monsanto's coalition has been whispering in their ear.

Not surprisingly, the Dairy Coalition memorandum also identified the International Dairy Foods Association as an "allied organization." Specifically, it noted:

> "A representative participated in a telephone conference call, per International Dairy Foods Association (IDFA's) request, to discuss strategy with the Grocery Manufacturers Association

(GMA) and the National Food Processors Association (NFPA), among others."[54]

In the memorandum, the Dairy Coalition also boasted about the success of The Machine at the press conference:

> "Overall our strategy was to downplay milk's presence on the list of "Dirty Dozen" consumer products…Our strategy was successful. Out of 200 television and radio news reports from around the country, only four had expanded coverage of milk…Print media coverage was minimal, so far nothing has appeared yet in *The Washington Post*, *The New York Times* or in *USA Today* (we will continue monitoring). The stories filed by *Associated Press* and *Reuters* reporters contained commentaries from our spokespersons."[54]

If the medical associations that advise us on both diet and medical treatments are spouting industry-crafted talking points, can we trust their "expert" advice?

### SEASONING

**Swaying The Masses**

An article published in *JAMA* in 1990 encouraged health professionals to engage in the rBGH controversy by "reassuring the public" that rBGH is safe.[70] In the *JAMA* article, the authors concluded:

> "…health professionals can play an important role in reassuring the public about the safety of milk and refuting misstatements or misconceptions about BST."[104]

Who wrote this article? Two scientists, Dr. Daughaday and Dr. Barbano. They were not affiliated with the FDA. They were, however, reported to be "Monsanto consultants."[54]

### 7. Advertisement

In addition to controlling brand messaging through news outlets and medical associations, the Dairy Coalition extended to the advertising world. Do you remember the "Happy Cow" commercials that featured smiling California cows playing on push green grass? The tag line was "Great Cheese comes from Happy Cows. Happy Cows come from California." This "Happy Cow" campaign was a national success. It was heard on radio, seen on television, and branded on t-shirts and stuffed toys. Barbie even has her own "Happy Cow" outfit.[105] That campaign has Dairy Coalition written all over it.

The successful "Happy Cow" campaign was developed for the California Milk Advisory Board (CMAB), which is one of the largest commodity boards in the United States. According to their website, their sole purpose is brand messaging:

> "We here at the California Milk Advisory Board (CMAB)... exist for one purpose: to spread the word about the extraordinary dairy products made with Real California Milk."[106]

The CMAB is supervised by the California Department of Food and Agriculture. And, the California Department of Food and Agriculture is a member of the National Association of State Departments of Agriculture (NASDA), which is part of the Dairy Coalition. All roads appear to lead back to the Dairy Coalition, hence Monsanto's Machine.

What's really interesting is that the government chooses the CMAB board of directors, and supervises the activity of the board, including the programs they carry out.[106] That means the government was essentially in charge of the "Happy Cow" campaign, i.e. they pushed the rBGH milk on the public through marketing. But wait, it gets worse.

Who funds the CMAB? Dairy farmers fund the board, but it's not voluntary. The dairy farmers pay a tax on every pound of milk they produce.[106] What that really means is: You and I pay that tax when consuming products that are produced by those farmers.

If you think that's bad, do you remember the "Got Milk" campaign? It was part of the Milk Processors' Education Program, which is a government program that is monitored by the USDA. According to their website, they are "funded by the nation's milk processors, who are committed to increasing fluid milk consumption."[107] In other words, the processors tax that was used to fund the "Got Milk" campaign was passed on to the consumer.[108,109]

**In the end, the government figured out how to get us to pay for both the approval of a genetically engineered hormone and for the promotion of the potential disease-causing foods that the hormone creates.**

## The Current State Of rBGH

rBGH is still approved by the FDA, therefore it is still legal to use in dairy cows. Additionally:

- The FDA still does not require labeling of products that come from animals injected with rBGH.
- Nor do they require labeling of foods that come from experimental trials.
- The FDA has not approved a drug residue assay, which is required for third party verification of the safety of our milk.
- Consequently, consumers must take the word of the drug manufacturers and the FDA at face value.

Whatever happened to Monsanto? In October of 2008, it sold the rBGH drug to Eli Lilly for over $300 million.[110]

## Here They Go Again

Beef cattle in the U.S. have been subjected to growth hormones since 1954, thanks to Eli Lilly.[111] That was the year the FDA approved the use of DES (diethylstilbestrol) in cows. It was the first synthetic hormone used to promote growth in cows, and it was manufactured by Eli Lilly.[112]

DES was a huge hit when it first appeared on the market. Within 2 years of approval, "an estimated two-thirds of the nation's beef cattle were treated with DES."[113] Then, in 1979, the FDA "withdrew approval of DES for use in cattle," which took DES off the market.[112] Why would the FDA take such a popular product off the market?

Roughly 7 years *before* it was approved for use in cows, DES was approved for use in pregnant women to help prevent miscarriage. However, DES ended up causing cancer in females that were exposed to the drug while in the womb:

> "DES, used as a human fertility treatment, is documented to have caused grotesque cancers in the daughters of treated women."[88]

Did Eli Lilly and the FDA learn from this terrible mistake?

No.

Once DES was scrapped, Eli Lilly forged ahead and began manufacturing rBGH alongside Monsanto.

In a controversial move, the FDA would later approve rBGH in addition to six other growth-promoting hormones in beef cattle. Consequently, nearly every beef cow in the U.S. currently receives some combination of growth hormones.[112,113] Research shows that when the hormone-treated cows are slaughtered, "not all steroids have been metabolized or excreted; measurable levels are, in fact, present in muscle, fat, liver, kidney and other organs present in meat products."[114] Thus, the FDA has defined an "acceptable daily intake" (ADI) for each of the six drugs. In other words, the FDA has decided how much of each hormone they feel is okay for us to eat every day. How did they decide the level that is "safe" for us to eat?

According to a 2007 study published in *Human Reproduction*, there is no way to determine what levels, if any, are safe for humans because they have not been properly tested:

> "These ADIs are based on traditional toxicological testing, and the possible effects on human populations exposed to residues of anabolic sex hormones through meat consumption have never, to our knowledge, been studied."[112]

Think about it: **For over 60 years, Americans have eaten steroid hormones in their beef and the health consequences are unknown.** That means every time you bought a fast-food hamburger, you ate hormones. When you made Hamburger Helper® for your children, they ate hormones. When you packed beef jerky for that camping trip, you were feeding your family hormones. Unless you specifically bought beef that was labeled as "hormone free," we have all eaten these hormones and nobody knows the consequence for our long-term health. But, don't worry. The government is here to protect you.

The government decided that these six hormones are safe for you and your children to consume on a regular basis because they claim their drug residues are harmless to humans![51] Is this sounding familiar?

Both rBGH and these six steroids are growth hormone, so they are all used for economic gains. The U.S. approved both rBGH and these six hormones with limited data to support their use in our food supply and no data regarding the effect of the drug residues on human health. And, now we're back to the same claim made by the FDA that hormone drug residues don't hurt people. Meanwhile, the first growth hormone the FDA approved, DES, was taken off the market because it caused cancer in humans.

Here's the final piece of the puzzle that makes the rBGH and beef hormone stories match perfectly: These six growth hormones were approved in the U.S. but they were banned in Europe, just like rBGH. European scientists and the European Commission "…claim hormone-treated beef is potentially toxic and unsafe for human consumption."[51]

---

( SEASONING )

## A Mothers Influence
In 2007, a study published in the scientific journal *Human Reproduction* reported that children born to mothers who ate beef containing growth hormones had a 24.3% lower sperm concentration compared with children who were born to mothers who ate less beef. The more beef the mothers ate, the more fertility issues the male children had. For instance, sons born to "high beef consumers" had nearly 3 times the level of subfertility compared with sons born to women who consumed low levels of beef. According to the study, "Sperm concentration was not significantly related to mother's consumption of other meat or to the man's consumption of any meat." The authors concluded, "These data suggest that maternal beef consumption, and possibly xenobiotics [including growth hormones] in beef, may alter a man's testicular development in utero and adversely affect his reproductive capacity."[112] If you think this couldn't happen to your child or grandchild, think again. This study was conducted in the United States! They tested mothers from five different U.S. cities between 1999 and 2005.

---

## Whose Fault Is It?

According to the FDA, it's our fault, as consumers, for not providing companies with the necessary incentive to invest in safety measures:

> "…the lack of awareness and information about the [safety] risks suggests than an inefficiently low demand may exist for food products that are produced using adequate measures to prevent

foodborne illness, adulteration, or contamination. Because the demand for many manufactured or processed foods may not be sufficiently affected by safety considerations, incentives to invest in safety measures from farm to fork is diminished. Consequently, the market may not provide the incentives necessary for optimal food safety."[115]

## What You Can Do

Thanks to consumer awareness, rBGH has become "one of the most controversial food products in the world."[116] You can help stamp out rBGH by reading your food labels and speaking with your dollars:

- **When purchasing animal products**:
  - o Buy from a local farmer. Ask for a tour of the facility so you can attempt to verify that their cows are not treated with rBGH.
  - o When buying from a grocery store, instead of conventional, buy organic meat, milk, cheese, and butter.
  - o Buy dairy products sourced from countries like Europe, where rBGH is banned.
  - o Unless you buy beef that is labeled as free of added hormones, you are probably eating meat from cows that were treated with growth hormones. Check your labels. Look for wording such as: "Raised without added hormones" or "No hormones administered."
- **Move the market in your community**:
  - o Call or email your local supermarket and request they carry conventional products that don't contain milk from cows treated with rBGH. Major retailers, including Wal-Mart and Kroger, have already committed to going rBGH-free. Even the nation's largest dairy processor, Dean Foods, will not allow rBGH-milk to enter their facility in New Jersey.[117]
  - o Call or email your local hospitals and schools. Ask them to remove all rBGH products from their facility. Some hospitals and schools have already responded to consumer pressure by banning rBGH products.[118]
- **Stay informed:**
  - o Support *The Milkweed* by subscribing to their monthly newsletter. It's a great way to stay informed about our milk supply while supporting a publication that speaks the truth.

*The Milkweed* has no advertisers or sponsors. Consequently, there is no agenda, except for seeking the truth. (www.the milkweed.com)

## Take Home Message

The FDA approved the first genetically engineered hormone for use in our food supply in spite of the fact that:

- The scientific literature reports a connection between rBGH and cancer promotion.
- FDA scientists repeatedly warned that rBGH could put public health in danger.
- The GAO advised against approval.
- FDA regulations had to be changed in order to approve the drug.
- Two industry-sponsored rat studies were used as the primary evidence to support the safety of milk from rBGH cows for human consumption.
- Most other industrialized nations banned the use of rBGH.

My biggest issue with the rBGH story is that both the U.S. government and Monsanto eroded our freedom. By not informing the public that a genetically engineered hormone was released into our food supply, and not requiring labeling of experimental products, they took away our right to decide what we want to put in our own bodies. Then, they manipulated us into believing that milk from cows treated with rBGH is the same as milk from cows not treated with a genetically modified growth hormone. And, much of this manipulation was done with our own tax dollars!

It's time for a gut check. Let's ask ourselves a critical question: *Has the government earned my trust in this situation?*

## Moving Forward

The story of rBGH lifted my veil of unearned trust in government, industry, and "experts." It sparked a revolution inside my mind and my heart. The more I learned, the more I questioned everything about our food supply. It didn't take long to realize that rBGH was just the beginning. rBGH ushered in a revolutionary new age of food where more than half of all the food we eat would be *fundamentally* and *irreversibly* changed.[44,47] Consequently, our bodies would no longer recognize the foods we once ate as children. It happened right under our noses, and many of us didn't even know about it. Why?

Just like we saw in our rBGH story, both the government and industry didn't think we had the right to know.

CHAPTER 8

# GMOS

## *A Story Of Déjà Vu*

"In response to concern raised by our customers...we have decided to remove, as far as possible, genetically modified soy and maize (corn) from all food products served in our restaurant. We will continue to work with our suppliers to replace GM soy and maize with non-GM ingredients...We have taken the above steps to ensure that you, the customer, can feel confident in the food we serve."[1]

—This statement hung on the wall in the cafeteria
at Monsanto's UK headquarters (1999).

We eat foods, like corn and sugar, which are *fundamentally* different from what our parents and grandparents ate. They are different because our supply of food is becoming dependent on genetic engineering.

We now have genetically engineered[†] (GE) fruits, vegetables, and fish. These foods are not found in nature. Instead, they are made in a laboratory by adding genes from organisms, like bacteria, to our food. Many of these genetically engineered foods are already in your supermarket: Approximately 75% of all processed foods in the grocery store

---

† The terms genetically engineered (GE) and genetically modified (GM) are used interchangeably.

contain GE ingredients.[2,3] Most Americans eat GE food every day and don't even know it because, once again, there is no FDA requirement to label these products.[4,5] Chances are, you've eaten GE foods today.

That's a frightening realization because GE foods were created by a handful of corporations, approved without any long-term safety studies, and are largely untested and unregulated.[5]

Throughout our next story, you will discover many similarities between the approval of rBGH and the approval of GE foods. For instance, both were approved for us to eat based on:

- **Insufficient scientific data**
- **A change in government regulation to fit the needs of the product**
- **Intimidation**
- **Retribution**
- **The revolving door**

So, grab a bowl of GE, subsidized popcorn covered in butter containing synthetic chemicals on the GRAS list and sourced from cows treated with rBGH, and let's dive into our next story.

## What Are GMOs?

Every living organism is made up of DNA, which is organized into segments called genes. Those genes determine your eye color, height, skin color, and other traits that make you unique. Genetically modified organisms (GMOs) are plants, animals, or other organisms whose **genes have been permanently changed in a laboratory.** The genes have been changed in a way that cannot occur naturally through breeding.[6] For instance, scientists can take a gene from one species, such as a human, and put that gene into a completely different species, such as a pig.

The purpose of genetic engineering is to change a characteristic of that organism. For instance, in the 1980s, USDA scientists wanted to create a faster-growing pig. Since scientists knew that humans have a gene that promotes growth, they thought, "Maybe we can take the gene from humans that makes them grow and put it into a pig to make the pig grow faster." So, they added a human gene to the pig to make it produce growth hormone. When the piglets were born with the newly added human genes, one piglet had no genitals or anus, while some of the piglets couldn't even stand. Other piglets had renal disease, arthritis, and enlarged hearts.[7]

Still, scientists were not deterred. They have continued to genetically engineer other organisms, including:

- Cows that produce human breast milk.[8]
- Goats that produce spider protein, which can be used to make bulletproof vests.[9]
- Pigs combined with jellyfish genes to make their noses light up.[10]
- Fish that grow up to 300% faster than a natural fish.[11]
- Human organs grown inside pigs to create donor organs that are part-human, part-pig.[12]
- Animals engineered to be susceptible to cancer so scientists can test out new medical therapies in their laboratories.[13]

Scientists have been playing around with GMOs since the early 1970s, and now they are using this technology to create GE crops that end up on our dinner plate. Consequently, **most of the food we eat in America contains ingredients that are genetically engineered.**[3,4] That doesn't bother many people I know because they believe genetic engineering is similar to traditional crop breeding. And, since farmers have been using traditional crop breeding for thousands of years, how bad could genetic engineering really be?

That is an understandable misconception. After all, the goal of genetic engineering is the same as the goal of traditional crop breeding: To have the new generation express a desired trait. However, the methods used to achieve that goal are completely different.

Traditional crop breeding involves crossing or interbreeding two plants of the *same or closely related species*. This is done using natural propagation techniques, such as pollination. In addition, the selected traits are not new to the plant. They include traits such as higher yields, disease resistance, or drought tolerance. This type of breeding occurs in nature.

In contrast, genetic engineering is done in a laboratory. The process involves scientists transferring a gene from one organism (i.e. plant, animal, or microorganism) into a second organism. It introduces an entirely new trait, one that is foreign to that organism. This is something that cannot happen on its own. It cannot happen in nature.[14] In fact, scientists can actually insert genes from one species into a *completely different species*.

Let's take corn, for example. For most of history, humans were not directly involved in the propagation process. They picked the best-performing seeds from the season, saved them, and planted them the next season. New mixes of genes did occur, but it was accomplished through the natural process of pollination. Specifically, pollen passed from the male part of the plant to the female. That process occurred naturally through insect pollinators or the wind. Importantly, this type of breeding occurred between two corn plants, i.e. between the same species.

In contrast, today, **most of the corn grown in the U.S. has a bacterial gene added to it.** That gene is called *Bacillus thuringiensis,* or *Bt.* It causes the corn to make *Bt* toxin, which is a pesticide. During the process of genetic engineering, the *Bt* gene becomes part of the corn's DNA, which causes the corn to make the pesticide inside its own cells. In essence, corn becomes a pesticide factory with nearly every cell in the corn making toxins. Consequently, when an insect bites into the corn, it ingests the toxin, which kills the insect by rupturing its gut.[15] In theory, this is brilliantly innovative. But, we eat that corn too. **With every bite of corn, we literally ingest toxins.** Does that sound like a good idea to you?

It's not. For years, "experts" have assured us that *Bt* toxin couldn't harm humans because it can't bind to our guts. However, research is emerging that casts doubt on that assertion. It may, in fact, be possible for *Bt* toxin to bind to our gut![16–20] If that happens, viruses, bacteria and other potentially harmful toxins can leak into our bloodstream, potentially causing disease.[21]

As an added bonus, the genes of the *Bt* corn are permanently changed. We cannot change the corn back to what it was originally. Once genetically engineered, always genetically engineered. In addition, once GMOs are taken out of the laboratory and released into nature, it's out of our hands. Corn that is genetically engineered to make *Bt* toxin can pass that ability to its offspring.[14] It can even pollinate non-genetically engineered plants, which can turn the new plant into a GE plant. We cannot stop it. Consequently, **there are no recalls when it comes to genetically engineered crops.**

No matter how you look at it, **genetic engineering has fundamentally changed our food supply.** The corn we knew as children is gone. It's some new, strange variety that is a fusion between corn and bacteria. It might even be a new species. Should we even call it corn? After all, the name "corn" comes with an expectation that all the genes in that corn are genes that belong to corn. So, when bacterial genes are added to corn and it is still labeled as corn, isn't that false advertising?

Think about it: When plums were crossed with apricots, the new fruit was given a new name: pluot. When tangerines were crossed with grapefruit, they also got a new name: tangelo. We also have limequats, which are a cross between a lime and a kumquat. The list goes on and on. All these fruits were renamed even though they were simply bred with other fruits, using pollen. So, why doesn't corn get a new name since it is now a cross between bacteria and corn? That corn makes a bacterial toxin inside itself. So, wouldn't it be more transparent to give this new creation a new name, like bactocorn or cornteria or cornoxin?

Sadly, corn isn't the only food that has changed in our lifetime. The big push for increasing industrial food farming in the 21$^{st}$ century is GE crops. There are two main types of GE crops in our food supply:

1. Crops that are genetically engineered to resist disease or insects, as in the case of *Bt* corn.
2. Crops that are genetically engineered to resist herbicides, like glyphosate, which we will discuss shortly.

Both types of GE crops are currently grown in America, including the following:

- Soy (94% of all soy grown in the U.S. is GMO)[22]
- Corn (92% is GMO)[22]
- Cotton (93% is GMO)[22]
- Canola (90% is GMO)[23]
- Sugar beets (95% is GMO)[24]
- Hawaiian papaya (over 50% is GMO)[23]
- Zucchini and yellow squash (over 24,000 acres is GMO)[25]

Who's behind this fundamental change in our food supply?

Monsanto.

Monsanto gave us rBGH, a genetically engineered hormone, and now they are pushing genetically engineered food. Monsanto, along with other chemical companies, have figured out how to merge our food with the chemicals they have created. Looking back, this was an obvious evolution because the chemical companies that make GMOs are the same companies (or their successors) that previously gave us pesticides, DDT, Agent Orange, PCBs, and dioxin. All of these chemicals are linked to cancer.[14] And now, these same chemical companies are making our food. That bears repeating: **Chemical companies are now creating our food.**

Chemical companies have brought us a new era of food, one where they play the role of God. By moving selected genes across species lines, they have broken the laws of nature. Species were designed to reproduce within their own kind, or within closely related species. And now, that fundamental law of nature has been thrown out the window. What could possibly go wrong?

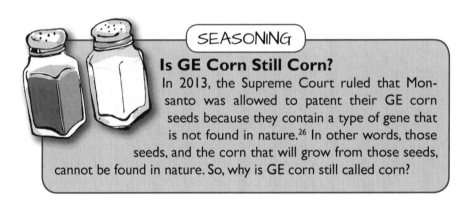

## SEASONING
### Is GE Corn Still Corn?
In 2013, the Supreme Court ruled that Monsanto was allowed to patent their GE corn seeds because they contain a type of gene that is not found in nature.[26] In other words, those seeds, and the corn that will grow from those seeds, cannot be found in nature. So, why is GE corn still called corn?

## SEASONING
### *Bt* Toxin On Organic Food
*Bt* toxin is used in organic farming to kill insects. *Bt* toxin, which is a crystal protein made by bacteria, is applied to organic plants. Sometimes, dead or weakened bacteria are applied as well. Once an insect eats the bacteria, it become active inside the gut of the insect and leads to death. However, if an insect doesn't eat the bacteria, it degrades in less than a day and can be washed off with water before you eat it. This is a different mechanism than what occurs with GE *Bt* corn. GE corn makes *Bt* toxins inside its' own cells. That toxin cannot be washed off, so we end up eating it.[27,28]

## Unintended Consequence: Sick Plants

Studies show that some GE crops are inferior to non-GE crops. For instance, some herbicide-resistant GE crops are more susceptible to disease, have weakened defenses, and suffer from reduced growth and vigor, according to a study in the *European Journal of Agronomy*.[29] In addition, deficiencies in manganese, copper, and zinc have been reported in GE crops.[29-32] Consequently, the plant can starve to death.

GE crops can also have inferior nutrient profiles compared with non-GE crops. For example, a study published in the *Journal of Medicinal Food* in 1999 reported a 12-14% lower concentration of phytoestrogen in GE soybeans compared with traditional soybeans.[33] That's bad because phytoestrogen is thought to help protect against heart disease.[34] In addition, a 2014 study published in *Food Chemistry* reported that organic soybeans have a better nutrient profile than GE soybeans. The study concluded:

> "Organic soybeans showed the healthiest nutritional profile with more sugars, such as glucose, fructose, sucrose and maltose, significantly more total protein, zinc and less fibre [fiber] than both conventional and GM-soy. Organic soybeans also contained less total saturated fat and total omega-6 fatty acids than both conventional and GM-soy."[30]

The bottom line is that GE plants are likely sicker than non-GE plants. Guess who eats the sick plants?

## Unintended Consequence: Sick Animals

Sick GE plants are fed to most of the livestock in the United States. In fact, their diet consists primarily of GMOs.[36,37] As a result, some livestock are getting sicker. For instance, sterility in both cows and pigs fed *Bt* corn has been reported in North America. In India, thousands of sheep and goats reportedly died shortly after eating *Bt* cotton plants.[38] In addition, cows, horses, and chickens in Asia reportedly died after eating *Bt* corn.[39]

These illnesses and deaths are not surprising. Scientific studies have reported serious health risks in animals that are fed GMOs, including:

- Reproductive Issues including Infertility[40-43]
- Increased Infant Mortality[44-46]

- Liver Damage[47–51]
- Impaired Digestion[48,52,53]
- Damaged Gastrointestinal System[54,55]
- Intestinal Cell Growth (possibly precancerous)[55,56]
- Activated Immune Response[57,58]
- Impaired Immune Function[54,59]

## SEASONING

### Why Would Farmers Buy GE Seeds?

Bt corn was supposed to save farmers money and help the environment by not requiring as much pesticide to be sprayed on the GE corn, compared to non-GE corn. Initially, that's exactly what happened. Insecticide application dropped by 123 million pounds between 1996 and 2011.[35] However, some of the major insects that infect Bt corn are growing resistant to the toxin it produces. Consequently, insecticide use has increased. Meanwhile, herbicide-resistant crops, such as Roundup Ready® corn, were supposed to decrease herbicide use. However, between 1996 and 2011, herbicide use on GE crops increased by 527 million pounds. Overall, between 1996 and 2011, as more GE crops were planted in the United States, pesticide use increased a total of 7% (404 million pounds).[35]

According to the American Academy of Environmental Medicine, the relationship between GMOs and disease is so strong that they declared GMOs to *cause* disease in animals. That's a huge deal! To claim something causes disease, the evidence has to be strong, consistent, specific, and likely to happen in the body. There is enough causal evidence that the American Academy of Environmental Medicine has called for a moratorium on GM foods.[60]

Even animals must know that GE plants are inferior in quality because there is evidence that, when given an option, they choose non-GE plants. In *Seeds of Deception*, Jeffrey Smith reported that in 1999, cows chose to eat non-GE plants instead of GE plants. Apparently, the cows didn't want to eat Roundup® Ready corn, so they broke through a fence to get to the non-GE corn.[61]

Clearly, eating sick plants has made animals sick. Guess who eats both the sick plants and the sick animals?

## Unintended Consequence: Sick People

We eat the sick plants and the sick animals. This suggests that we are likely to become sick as well.

Available evidence[‡] supports a connection between consuming GMOs (sometimes in relation to the chemicals sprayed on those foods) and impaired health in humans, including:

- Cellular damage that could lead to Inflammatory Diseases such as Alzheimer's, Autism, and Heart Disease.[62]
- Breast Cancer[63]
- Endocrine Disruption[64]
- DNA Damage[62,65]
- Allergies[66,67]

Keep in mind that many of the diseases I've mentioned don't appear until years after you have been consuming the chemical culprit. There is a cumulative effect. So, you might feel perfectly fine for years, but GM foods may get you in the long run. For example, in 1999, the medical journal *Cancer* reported an increased risk of non-Hodgkin's Lymphoma in humans exposed to glyphosate, a chemical used on approximately 80% of GM crops.[62,68] Furthermore, the study revealed, "the highest [cancer] risks were seen when first exposure occurred 10-20 years before diagnosis."[68] That's bad news for us because a record level of glyphosate has been sprayed on our food since the introduction of GMOs, roughly 20 years ago.[69]

Having said that, the potential health consequences that stem from GMOs are a complicated and controversial subject that requires many more pages than what I can dedicate in this book. In preparing to write this chapter, I conducted extensive research on this topic. What I found led me to take my family off GMOs. I encourage you to do your own homework

---

‡ For a detailed analysis of the association between GMOs and disease, I recommend reading Jeffrey Smith's books titled, *Genetic Roulette: The Documented Health Risks of Genetically Engineered Foods* and *Seeds of Deception: Exposing Industry and Government Lies about the Safety of the Genetically Engineered Foods You're Eating.*

and decide for yourself if GMOs are right for *your* family. I've provided references to get you started.

But, we don't have to agree that GMOs are harmful. "Proving" that GMOs are bad is not the point of this book. I'm more interested in the fact that the FDA has perpetuated the veil of unearned trust by providing an illusion that the agency has "safety" tested and "approved" of GMOs.

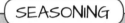

SEASONING

## Bad Day for Allergic Reactions

The process of genetic engineering intentionally introduces new proteins into the plant. However, there is a risk that unknown proteins are introduced during the process as well. Proteins can cause allergic reactions. Yet, there are no government guidelines for how to assess the potential of allergic reactions to GM foods.[70] Even if our government did require testing for allergenicity, it would be futile because we don't currently have a way to test for which proteins are present in GM foods. How do you test for a protein that you don't know exists?[14]

## Changing Regulations To Suit Industry

If you recall, the use of rBGH in cows led to increased disease, which required treatment with antibiotics. The antibiotic use increased so much that the level of antibiotic residue in the milk was higher than the FDA allowed. The FDA changed its own regulation in order to approve the first genetically engineered hormone in our food supply.[61] A similar situation occurred with the "approval" of GMOs.

Roundup Ready® soybeans, the first successfully bioengineered crop, were introduced in the United States in 1996. Roundup Ready® soybeans are genetically engineered to tolerate Roundup®. You've probably heard of Roundup®. It's the weed killer people commonly spray on their yards. It's also used on food crops. In the case of Roundup Ready® soybeans, the soy is genetically modified so that it can tolerate exposure to Roundup®. Specifically, the soybean isn't killed when glyphosate, the herbicide in Roundup®, touches it.[30] In theory, Roundup® can be sprayed on the soybean crops to kill weeds without hurting the genetically modified soybean plant.

Roundup Ready® soybeans are a brilliant business model because the GM seeds and Roundup® go hand in hand, like peanut butter and jelly. The farmer *must* use them together.[30] If farmers use a different herbicide, one that does not contain glyphosate, the GM soybeans will likely be killed because they have been modified to tolerate Roundup®, specifically glyphosate. Guess which company makes both the GM seeds and Roundup®?

Monsanto.

Thus, farmers are incentivized to buy both their seeds and their herbicide from Monsanto. In fact, companies other than Monsanto sell glyphosate-based herbicides. But, Monsanto has a licensing agreement that does not allow farmers who plant Roundup Ready® crops to use any glyphosate-based product other than Roundup®.

That business model has been wildly successful. For instance, 94% of U.S. soy is genetically engineered to be Roundup Ready®.[22] And, in 2014, Roundup Ready® soy was the number one GM crop in the *world*. Since the technology only works with glyphosate, it's no surprise that glyphosate was the most widely used herbicide in the world that same year. Consequently, the vast majority of soy is now genetically modified *and* treated with Roundup®.[30]

There's only one small problem: Weeds became resistant to the glyphosate in Roundup®.[71]

Monsanto assured farmers that weed resistance would not be a problem.[72] Nonetheless, superweeds have developed, which means farmers have incurred increased weed management costs, sometimes as high as 50-100%.[71] Some of that cost stems from the need to spray more glyphosate on crops to keep the weeds at bay. Consequently, more glyphosate is sprayed on our food than ever before:

- Glyphosate has been sprayed on crops since the mid-1970s, yet 74% of all the glyphosate ever used in the U.S. has been sprayed in the last 10 years.[73]
- For comparison, roughly 11 million pounds of Roundup® were used in 1987 while nearly 300 million pounds were sprayed on our crops in 2015.[74]

- Glyphosate has been used so extensively in the U.S. that it is now found in 75% of air and rain samples.[75]
- Worldwide, enough glyphosate has been sprayed to cover every single cultivated acre of land with roughly half a pound of Roundup®.[74]

Consequently, "extreme levels" of Roundup® (i.e. glyphosate) have been detected on GE soy, as reported in the scientific journal *Food Chemistry* in 2014.[30] 70% of the GE-soy samples that were tested contained glyphosate residue levels that Monsanto itself defined as "extreme."[30] We eat that soy in our processed foods, some of us on a daily basis, and now we are learning that it can contain "extreme" levels of a chemical that the World Health Organization declared to be "probably carcinogenic to humans."[65] That means **glyphosate likely causes cancer**. In addition, studies have shown glyphosate to be associated with birth defects, DNA damage, and other health problems.[68,76,77] But, *we* have nothing to worry about because surely the government monitors the amount of glyphosate on our food and would tell us if we were eating "extreme" levels of a probable cancer-causing agent, right?

Wrong.

High levels of glyphosate can be a problem for plant, animal, and human health. That's why the EPA sets a limit for the amount of glyphosate residue allowed on our food. After Roundup Ready® soybeans were on the market, the legal limit was raised to 20 mg/kg. Why?

**The U.S. government changed its regulation so GM crops could continue to be sold.[78,79]**

The amount of glyphosate sprayed on GM crops, like Roundup Ready® soybeans, increased as the herbicide technology failed. Consequently, GM soybeans contained more glyphosate than allowed, so the rules had to be changed to allow the continued sale of GM soybeans.[78,79] Just as we saw in our rBGH story, regulations were changed to fit the product instead of the product being modified or improved to adhere to existing regulations.

It's time for a gut check: Has the government earned your trust in this situation?

## How Much GMO And Glyphosate Do You Eat?

If you recall from our farm subsidies story, Americans are predominately GM "corn chips" with a dollop of GM soy on top.[81] That's because the average American eats roughly 75% of their calories from subsidized, processed foods and approximately 75% of those foods contain GMOs.[2,3] In fact, GMOs are so abundant in our diet that the **average adult eats *at least* 200 pounds of GMOs every year,** according to the Environmental Working Group.[82]

Even our babies eat GMOs. Nearly all infant formulas contain GMOs, either in the form of milk from cows that were treated with the genetically engineered bovine growth hormone or as derivatives of GM corn or GM soy.[83] The U.S. government provides free formula to roughly 2 million babies, and almost all of it contains GMOs.[84]

In terms of Roundup®, an estimated **93% of Americans have glyphosate in their bodies**, with children having the highest level, according to a study conducted by the University of California San Francisco in 2015.[85] In addition, pesticides associated with GM crops have been found in the blood of pregnant women and their unborn babies.[86] That's alarming since those types of chemicals affect babies and children at smaller doses than adults, putting them at greater risk for associated health issues.[87,88]

The bottom line is: Most **babies, children, and adults in America eat GMOs and Roundup® every day**. And, most of us don't realize it. But, I'm sure we have nothing to worry about. After all, *someone* in the government has checked them for safety, right?

## GMOs Are GRAS

Do you remember the GRAS list? It is the list of chemicals allowed in our food that are not safety checked or regulated by the FDA. Instead, companies determine if their chemicals are safe and then the companies regulate themselves. Guess what made it on the GRAS list?

GE crops!

All GE crops and all GM foods made from those crops are "presumed" to be GRAS by the FDA.[5] Remember when I told you that approximately 75% of all processed food contains GMOs? All of those GM ingredients that you eat, probably *every day*, are GRAS.[5]

Since they are GRAS, the FDA relies "almost exclusively" on industry to make sure GM crops and GM foods are safe. According to the FDA, **"Ultimately, it is the food producer who is responsible for assuring safety."**[5]

Consequently, industry has been given a free pass to grow and sell GE crops and GM food without any "red tape." From the chemistry laboratory where scientists create the GE seeds to the grocery store shelves where GMOs end up in our favorite cookies and cakes, there is:

- **No regulation**
- **No oversight**
- **No FDA labeling requirement**
- **No requirement to notify the FDA** when a company puts a new GM food on the market.[5]
- **No requirement to conduct long-term safety testing**

What is the consequence of not requiring long-term safety studies on GM foods?

**We, the consumers, are the long-term study.**

Once again, you and I have been offered up as guinea pigs. And, since GM foods are relatively new, we won't know the long-term consequences of eating GMOs until well into the future. Even then, it will be difficult to determine a cause and effect relationship since there are no FDA labeling requirements.[5] After all, **Americans have been consuming GM food for roughly 20 years and most of us don't even know it.** How can we determine the effect of genetically modified foods on our health if we don't know when we are eating them?

We can't.

Without labeling, we can't track who is eating GM foods and how much they are eating. Consequently, it's nearly impossible to prove cause and effect and to, subsequently, sue industry for damages. The former EPA Medical Science Advisor, Dr. Lawrence Plumlee, believes this is intentional. According to Dr. Plumlee:

> "We're all part of a large uncontrolled experiment and we aren't getting answers because we don't know who's eating genetically engineered food and who isn't. So we have no way to do the studies. I suspect that this is the intention of the manufacturer. Let's so confuse the situation that no liability could ever be ascertained even if there is a big problem."[83]

Additionally, because GM foods are GRAS, **our voice is largely silenced.** The FDA offers a public comment period when an additive is undergoing a safety review. But if a chemical is GRAS, there is no public comment period.[90] Therefore, new products containing GMOs can end up on our dinner plate without us knowing and without us being included in the review process.

## GMOs Are Illegal

In 1958, Congress declared that a substance could be considered GRAS if that substance met two requirements:

1. Recognized as safe based on a consensus of "experts."
2. Recognized as safe based on "scientific procedures," which entails peer-reviewed scientific studies.[93]

"Genetically engineered (GE) foods fail both requirements,"[94] according to Steven Druker, founder of the Alliance for Bio-Integrity.

On May 27, 1998, Steven Druker filed a lawsuit challenging the FDA policy on GMOs. That lawsuit forced FDA records to be made public, which revealed the truth. According to Mr. Druker, the records prove there is no scientific consensus on the safety of GMOs, and the FDA has been lying to us:

> "[The records] revealed that politically appointed administrators had covered up the extensive warnings of their own scientists about the unusual risks of these foods, lied about the facts, and then ushered these novel products onto the market in violation of explicit mandates of federal food safety law. [94,95]

The declassified FDA records revealed that FDA scientists openly disagreed with the FDA policy on GMOs:

- Dr. Linda Kahl wrote a memo to the FDA Biotechnology Coordinator James Maryanski in 1992 stating, "The process of genetic engineering and traditional breeding are different, and according to the technical experts in the agency, they lead to different risks."[96]
- FDA microbiologist, Dr. Louis Pribyl, commented that a draft of the FDA policy "reads very proindustry, especially in the area of unintended effects…There is a profound difference between the types of unexpected effects from traditional breeding and genetic engineering which is just glanced over in this document…This is industry's pet idea, namely that there are no unintended effects that will raise the FDA's level of concern. But time and time again, there is no data to back up their contention."[97]
- Dr. E.J. Matthews worked in the FDA's Toxicology Group. He warned that "genetically modified plants could…contain unexpected high concentrations of plant toxicants."[98]
- The Director of the FDA's Center for Veterinary Medicine said, "CVM believes that animal feeds derived from genetically modified plants present unique animal and food safety concerns."[99]

In 1992, the FDA published a food policy document that provides evidence to support the concerns of the FDA scientists. In that document, the FDA recognized that genetic modification of crops can "introduce a protein that differs significantly in structure or function, or…modify a carbohydrate, fat or oil, such that it differs significantly in composition from such substances currently found in food."[5] In addition, the FDA recognized that GM crops might introduce new allergens into our food supply:

> "All food allergens are proteins…FDA's principal concern regarding allergenicity is that proteins transferred from one food source to another, as is possible with recombinant DNA… might confer on food from the host plant the allergenic properties of food from the donor plant. Thus, for example, the introduction of a gene that encodes a peanut allergen into corn might make that variety of corn newly allergenic to people ordinarily allergic to peanuts."[5]

In addition, the lack of consensus among "experts" isn't isolated to the FDA. For example:

- *The Lancet*, a respected medical journal, stated there is "good reason to believe that specific risks may exists [with GMOs]" and "governments should never have allowed these products into the food chain without insisting on rigorous testing for effects on health."[100]
- The Royal Society of Canada declared that the "default presumption" for all GMOs should be that unintended and potentially harmful side effects have been introduced into these foods.[101]
- The British Medical Association stated, "more research is needed to show that genetically modified (GM) food crops and ingredients are safe for people and the environment and that they offer real benefits over traditionally grown foods."[102]
- In 2013, the Public Health Association of Australia called for "an immediate and indefinite freeze" on growing GM crops.[103]
- In 2009, a review of the available toxicology studies on GMOs concluded that "most" of the studies indicated GMOs "may cause hepatic, pancreatic, renal, and reproductive effects and may alter hematological, biochemical, and immunological parameters, the significance of which remains unknown."[104]
- More than 300 scientists signed a statement in January of 2015 declaring there is no consensus regarding the safety of GMOs.[105]

"This lack of consensus in itself disqualified GE foods from GRAS status," according to Mr. Druker.[106] Perhaps that's why the safety concerns of scientists working at the FDA were allegedly covered up. Guess who was in charge of food safety at that time?

Michael Taylor.

Remember him? Mr. Taylor helped get rBGH-milk on the market. He was instrumental in crafting the disclaimer on my milk label, which stated no difference between rBGH-milk and milk from cows not treated with hormones. Likewise, Mr. Taylor was also instrumental in crafting the FDA's GMO policy that unleashed GMOs into our food supply with no long-term testing, no government regulation, and no oversight.[107]

Mr. Taylor's involvement may partly explain why Dr. James Maryanski, the former Biotechnology Coordinator at the FDA, declared the government policy on GMOs to be based on politics:

"It was a political decision. It was a very broad decision that didn't just apply to foods. It applied to all products of biotechnology."[108]

Let that sink in: The man in charge of biotechnology at the FDA told us that **the lack of regulation of all GMO products was based on politics** and not science.

Further evidence to support his claim lies in a memo from an FDA official to the Biotechnology Coordinator. In that memo, the FDA official queried, "are we asking the scientific experts to generate the basis for this policy statement in the absence of any data?"[109] That memo was contained within the FDA files that Mr. Druker was able to obtain. It demonstrates that as of 1992, when the FDA policy on GMOs was crafted, "there was virtually no evidence to support safety."[94]

Not only was the GMO policy of the FDA based on politics, according to Mr. Druker, **the FDA policy is illegal:**[§]

"There is substantial dispute among experts about their safety, and their safety has not been established through adequate testing…the FDA has been illegally, and fraudulently, exempting

---

§ For a detailed account of "the biggest scientific fraud of our age," I recommend reading *Altered Genes, Twisted Truth* by Steven Druker. Jane Goodall hailed it as "without a doubt one of the most important books of the last 50 years."

GE foods from the testing requirements established by Congress in 1958…the FDA's policy on GE foods violates the law, and those foods have entered the market illegally."[94]

### SEASONING

### The Hunger Myth
Monsanto claims that GM food could end world hunger. They even ran advertisements claiming, "Biotechnology is one of tomorrow's tools in our hands today. Slowing its acceptance is a luxury our hungry world cannot afford."[112] World hunger is not caused from lack of food production. According to the World Food Programme, the largest humanitarian agency in the world fighting hunger, "The world produces enough to feed the entire global population of 7 billion people."[113] It estimates that one-third of all the food produced is never consumed; we waste it.

## A Dream Of The Past

Looking through the scientific literature, you will find studies published in reputable journals that promote the safety of GMOs. However, I encourage you to check the affiliations of the scientists who conducted those studies.

A cozy relationship has developed between industry and universities. For instance, industry pays universities to conduct research on their products. Scientists are paid by industry through corporate-endowed positions. Professors can own stock in the same companies that sponsor their research. And, scientists are paid by industry to sit on their advisory boards. This crony relationship has created a new era of research where study outcomes overwhelmingly fall in industry's favor. You don't need to look further than aspartame for supporting evidence.

The sweetener aspartame, marketed under the name NutraSweet®, was extensively studied by 1995. Nearly 165 peer-reviewed studies looked at its safety. Roughly half of the studies found no problems associated with using aspartame. 100% of those studies were funded by the manufacturer.[114] In contrast, 92% of the studies funded by independent entities found problems with aspartame.[114] Can you guess who manufactured aspartame?

The manufacturer of aspartame was GD Searle, which was a subsidiary of Monsanto at that time.[61]

And, by the way, aspartame is genetically engineered.

Like universities, government has formed a partnership with industry. For instance, the USDA jointly owns over 150 U.S. agricultural biotechnology patents granted from 1982 to 2001, which include GMO patents.[115] That means the USDA collects royalties on GMOs! Clearly, the USDA is not impartial. The government is incentivized to help universities and industry push GM crops to market.

While none of these cozy relationships are illegal, they certainly introduce bias. Can we trust the findings of a study that was conducted by scientists who are on the industry payroll, and funded by the very same people who have a large incentive to get their product to market?

Clearly, the relationship between science, industry, and government has been blurred. There is no true objectivity. In an editorial published in *Physicians and Scientists for Responsible Application of Science and Technology*, Dr. Jaan Suurkula wrote:

"Scientific experts cannot be expected to be independent and reliable advisors in safety issues considering the increasing dependence of science on financial support from the industry."[116]

**Independent science is a dream of the past.** Say hello to the new age of "experts" for hire.

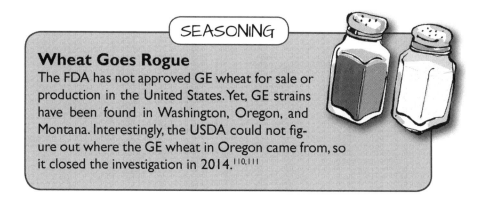

SEASONING

**Wheat Goes Rogue**
The FDA has not approved GE wheat for sale or production in the United States. Yet, GE strains have been found in Washington, Oregon, and Montana. Interestingly, the USDA could not figure out where the GE wheat in Oregon came from, so it closed the investigation in 2014.[110,111]

## Intimidation

There are a handful of scientists who have remained trustworthy by conducting independent research in pursuit of truth, instead of an agenda. Unfortunately, scientists who have the courage to speak the truth about GMOs are often intimidated and reprimanded. Here are just a few examples that were brought to light by Jeffrey Smith and Steven Druker:

- Dr. Elaine Ingham was a Soil Microbiologist at Oregon State University. After reporting on the dangers of GMOs at an international conference, she was scolded by the department head. Then, the former President of the University sent a letter stating that any bioscience faculty member that did not support genetic engineering didn't belong at Oregon State University.[117]
- Dr. Ignacio Chapela was working at UC Berkeley when he discovered that GM corn from the United States had contaminated the non-GM corn crops in Mexico. After publishing his findings in *Nature*, he was threatened, denied tenure, and a campaign was organized to discredit him.[83] *Nature* retracted part of Dr. Chapela's article. Two weeks later, the Mexican government confirmed that their corn crops were contaminated.
- Dr. Irina Ermakova, a senior scientist from the Russian National Academy of Sciences, reported that when female rats ate GM soy that was purchased at a grocery store, over half of their offspring died. She was publicly attacked, discredited, and ordered to stop conducting research on GM foods.[118]

Even the former Secretary of Agriculture, Dan Glickman, was reprimanded for suggesting the government think through the GMO issue. He served under Bill Clinton from 1995-2000, which means he was the acting Secretary when Round-up Ready® soybeans were introduced in the United States in 1996. According to Mr. Glickman, the sentiment inside the government was 'either you are with us or against us':

"What I found in the early years I was involved in the regulation of biotechnology was there was a general feeling in agribusiness and inside our government in the U.S. that if you weren't marching lockstep forward in favor of rapid approvals of biotech products, rapid approval of GMO crops, then somehow you were anti-science and anti-progress."[83]

When Mr. Glickman did speak out, he was "slapped around." According to Mr. Glickman:

"I would say even when I opened my mouth in the Clinton administration I got slapped around a little bit by not only the industry but also some of the people even in the administration. In fact, I made a speech once saying we needed to more thoughtfully think through the GMO issues and I had some people within the Clinton administration, particularly in the U.S. Trade area, that were very upset with me. They said, 'How could you in agriculture be questioning our regulatory regime?'"[83]

If our Secretary of Agriculture felt that type of immense pressure, imagine how difficult it was for a scientist working for the government to speak out against GMOs. One scientist did speak out, early in the GMO revolution, and he paid a steep price.

Dr. Arpad Pusztai worked for the Rowett Institute in Aberdeen, Scotland, for 30 years. He lost his job when he warned the public about the potential dangers of GM foods. His story began in 1995, when he was chosen to create a scientific protocol that could be used to verify the safety of GMOs. His protocol was supposed to become the European standard for testing GM food safety. There were no published studies on the safety of GM foods at that time. Dr. Pusztais' would be the first.[83] Keep in mind that we, in the U.S., were already consuming GM foods.

While working on his protocol, Dr. Pusztai was asked by the Rowett Institute director to review data that was submitted from various biotech companies. These companies were seeking approval of their GM soy, corn, and tomatoes. While reading through the 700 pages of documents submitted by the biotech companies, Dr. Pusztai realized that the evidence to support GMOs was flimsy and weak. According to Dr. Pusztai:

"As a scientist, I was really shocked. This was the first time I realized what flimsy evidence was being presented to the committee. There was missing data, poor research design, and very superficial tests indeed. Theirs was a very unconvincing case. And, some of the work was really very poorly done. I want to impress on you, it was a real shock."[61]

Consequently, Dr. Pusztai did not recommend approval. Much to his surprise, his approval wasn't needed. *GM foods had already been approved 2 years earlier.* The director wanted Dr. Pusztai to find a scientific basis for approval. After all, Dr. Pusztai and millions of people living in the UK had been unknowingly eating GM soy, corn, and tomatoes for nearly 2 years.[61] Apparently the U.S. isn't the only country that uses its citizens as un-consenting guinea pigs.

In the meantime, Dr. Pusztai was still responsible for creating the protocol that would determine if GMOs were safe. Dr. Pusztai and his team were testing potatoes that were genetically modified to resist aphids. They tested the effects of the GM potato on rats. The study revealed that the nutrient profile of the GM potatoes was different than the non-GM potato. For example, one GM potato had 20% less protein.[61]

In addition, the GM potato caused inflammation by activating the immune system of the rats. Compared to rats that ate non-GM potato, rats that ate GM potato had smaller brains, livers, and testicles as well as enlarged tissues, including the pancreas and intestines. There was also cell growth in the stomach and intestines, which could lead to tumors or cancer.[61] Based on the data, it was clear to Dr. Pusztai that GM foods were potentially harmful to humans. He was holding the evidence in his hands. He knew millions of people were already eating the GM food. What should he do?

What would you do? Would you stand up to the government by warning people that the food they are eating could make them sick? Or, would you keep quiet and save your job, along with your reputation?

Dr. Pusztai didn't have long to think about that moral dilemma; he was quickly put to the test. Dr. Pusztai was asked to do an interview for the British TV show "World in Action." On August 10, 1998, during his interview, Dr. Pusztai stated, "As a scientist actively working on the field, I find it is very, very unfair to use our fellow citizens as guinea pigs." Pusztai's statement made headlines throughout Europe. People became fearful of what the government was doing to their food supply.

Shortly after, Dr. Pusztai was forced to retire. By August 20th, 10 days after his TV interview, Dr. Pusztai was under a gag order. His research team was dismantled. Dr. Stanley Ewen from the University of Abderdeen, who was a collaborator of Dr. Pusztai, was forced to retire and was also discredited. Later, he learned he was fired because of a phone call. Dr. Ewen recalls, "Some pressure [was] being put on Tony

Blaire's office to stop this work because it was perceived by Americans to be harming their industrial base, the biotech industry in other words."[83] Who was on the phone call?

The British press reported that Tony Blair was the recipient of the phone call. The caller was alleged to be **President Bill Clinton** who was nudging Tony Blaire to support GMOs.[119]

Dr. Pusztai and his collaborators are martyrs for letting people know what the government and industry did to the food supply. Their bravery sparked consumer rejection of GMOs in Great Britain and parts of Western Europe. The media helped by spreading the word: Over 700 articles on GMOs were printed in just one month in Great Britain.[120] By April of 1999, the consumers united voice had been heard loud and clear. The European Union passed a law requiring any food containing more than 1 percent GMOs to be labeled. To avoid labeling, many European manufacturers simply eliminated GM ingredients. Nestle, McDonald's, Burger King, and some supermarkets, including Safeway and Somerfield, jumped on the non-GMO bandwagon.[61] Those companies responded to the market; they responded to the demands of the people. Did those companies remove GMOs from our food, here in the United States?

No!

Because "We the People of the United States" did not push back like the people did in parts of Europe and Great Britain.

## Media Goes Dark

What did America do during the Pusztai scandal and the subsequent grassroots uprising of the people in Great Britain and parts of Europe?

We were mostly silent even though we were already eating GMOs.

By this time, America already had GM potatoes, corn, soybeans, canola, and cottonseed oil (mainly used for frying foods), yet the U.S. media largely ignored the topic of GMOs.[121] Project Censored, a media watchdog group, listed GMOs as one of the top 25 most underreported events of the year.[122] Did you know you were eating GMOs back in 1999?

I certainly didn't.

## Labeling War

I didn't know I was eating GMOs until I read my milk label. The disclaimer on that label is how I found out about rBGH. Without that disclaimer, I would still be in the dark with a thick veil over my eyes, and this book would not exist.

GE crops and GM foods in America are not required by the FDA to carry a label even though 90% of Americans want genetically modified foods to be labeled.[123] Consequently, we've been in the dark for over twenty years. Meanwhile, over sixty countries require labeling of GM foods, including most industrialized nations. Even China requires labeling.[5,124]

It's possible that we are more in the dark today than ever before when it comes to knowing which foods are genetically engineered because of the "Deny Americans the Right to Know (DARK) Act," officially known as the Safe and Accurate Food Labeling Act. The DARK Act is a bill that was passed by Congress and signed into law by President Obama on July 29th, 2016. It was sold as a federal mandate requiring all products containing GMOs to be labeled, but it's filled with loopholes. For instance, most processed foods will not be required to be labeled as GMO, according to the Institute for Responsible Technology. In addition, for those foods that do qualify, companies don't have to use the word "GMO" on the label. Instead, they can provide an 800 number or a QR code, which would require consumers to hunt down the information. Not surprisingly, companies can ignore the new law without any penalty because there is currently no enforcement in place, according to the Institute for Responsible Technology.[125]

In addition, the DARK Act took away states' rights. That one bill placed the decision of labeling in the hands of the federal government with little recourse for the states or the people. For example, Vermont passed a law requiring all GMO products sold in their state to be labeled. That law went into effect on July 1, 2016. Twenty-eight days later, the DARK Act was passed, which swooped in and crushed it. Federal law preempts state law, so Vermont's GMO labeling law was voided. Personally, I'm against mandatory labeling. I choose to support third party verification groups, which we will discuss in Chapter 11.

The most troubling aspect of the DARK Act is that it may have created a veil around the issue of GMOs. Think about it: Lawmakers can say they did their job by cracking down on the food industry. And, the food industry can say it is following the federal law in terms of labeling their products as GMO. Consequently, this new law might provide consumers with a false sense of security; thereby lulling them back to sleep. If we're not careful, it could be 1906 all over again, when the veil first fell over our eyes.

## The Free Market Wins Again!

Campbell's® voluntarily pledged to label their products containing GMOs. In 2016, Campbell's® posted encouraging words for free market supporters on their website:

"We are operating with a 'Consumer First' mindset. We put the consumer at the center of everything we do. That's how we've built trust for nearly 150 years. We have always believed that consumers have the right to know what's in their food. GMO has evolved to be a top consumer food issue reaching a critical mass of 92% of consumers in favor of putting it on the label."[126]

Campbell's® also created a website (www.whatsinmyfood.com) that lists the ingredients in their products, and also indicates which ingredients might be genetically modified.[127]

## The Current State Of GMOs

As of 2015, a new option was added to our food menu. The FDA approved GE salmon for human consumption. It was the first GE animal approved for us to eat.[128] In addition, potatoes that don't bruise and apples that don't brown are on the horizon. Both have been "approved" for use in our food supply and both are expected to arrive on your grocery store shelf in the near future.[129]

But, there is good news! A study out of Italy suggests we can reverse the damage caused by GMOs. Scientists fed mice GM soybeans, which resulted in liver damage. Then, the same mice were placed on a non-GMO diet. The liver damage was reversed![130] We don't know the tipping point yet: We don't know how long you can eat GMOs before the damage is irreversible. However, this news brings much needed hope: Even though Americans have eaten GMOs for over 20 years, if damage has occurred, we might be able to reverse it, at least to some extent.

## What You Can Do

- **When buying processed food:**
  - Look for the Butterfly, which is the most trusted label available for GMO avoidance. The Butterfly belongs to the Non-GMO Project, which is a non-profit, independent organization dedicated to preserving and building the non-GMO food supply. We will discuss this option in more detail in Chapter 11.
  - Visit the Non-GMO Project's consumer website to find non-GMO verified alternatives to your favorite processed foods, including: breads, cereal, drinks, and more. (www.livingnongmo.org)
  - Grab a free copy of the Non-GMO Shopping Guide to help you identify foods containing GMOs in the grocery store. (www.responsibletechnology.org)
  - Look for the USDA Certified 100% Organic label. That seal means the food is not allowed to knowingly contain GMOs.
  - When buying corn, soy, and canola, choose organic.

- **When buying animal products:**
  - Choose organic meat, eggs, milk, cheese, butter, and yogurt that contain the Butterfly label.
  - Choose grass-fed beef as opposed to beef from animals fed GMOs.
- **Stay informed** by signing up for email alerts from leaders in the field, including:
  - *Institute for Responsible Technology:* A world leader in educating the public and policy makers about GM foods and crops, including associated health risks. (www.responsible technology.org)
  - *GM Watch:* A public news and information service that provides up-to-date and accurate information about genetically modified foods and crops. (www.gmwatch.org)
  - *Center for Food Safety:* A non-profit public interest and environmental advocacy organization that promotes organic and other sustainable agriculture. (www.centerforfood safety.org)
- **Donate** to organizations that fight to preserve the non-GMO food supply, such as:
  - The Non–GMO Project (www.nongmoproject.org)
  - Institute for Responsible Technology (www.responsible technology.org)
  - The Alliance for Bio-Integrity (www.biointegrity.org)
  - Center for Food Safety (www.centerforfoodsafety.org)

## Take Home Message

Today, most of our calories come from food that is fundamentally different than the food we ate as children. Corn is no longer corn. Soy is no longer soy. These foods have been co-opted by chemical companies who have permanently changed them into new varieties, or species, of food-like substances that don't exist in nature. Our bodies may have a difficult time recognizing and dealing with these new chemicals.[135] Consequently, they may be making us sicker.

But, we don't have to agree that GMOs are harmful to our health. Decide for yourself what is right for your family. However, when it comes to GMOs, I believe we can find common ground:

- Can we agree that the hands-off approach of the FDA puts our health in jeopardy?
- Can we agree that the FDA has perpetuated the veil of unearned trust by providing an illusion that the agency has safety tested and "approved" of GMOs?

By presuming GE crops and GM foods to be GRAS, there is practically no safety testing, toxicity testing, long-term testing, regulation, or monitoring by the FDA. In addition, industry gets to decide which genetically modified organisms will end up on your dinner plate. In the end, you and I are the ones that lose. We are the un-consenting guinea pigs, once again.

## Moving Forward

We've spent the last four chapters learning how the veil of unearned trust has allowed government, industry, and "experts" to fundamentally change our food supply. Now allow me to explain how they have fundamentally changed *you*. Most of us realize that industry tries to persuade us to buy certain foods through advertising and marketing. But, the government also nudges you to choose the foods they want you to eat. They've been doing it our entire lives, and many of us don't realize it. In the next chapter, we will explore how the government has fundamentally changed the way we *perceive* food and, in doing so, has helped separate us from our food and from ourselves.

CHAPTER 9:

# DIETARY GUIDELINES

## *The Pyramid Of Deception*

"A nudge, as we will use the term, is any aspect of the choice architecture that alters people's behavior in a predictable way without forbidding any options or significantly changing their economic incentives."

—Cass Sunstein and Richard Thaler, *Nudge: Improving Decisions about Health, Wealth, and Happiness*

In 1906, out of fear, Americans abdicated their role as watchdogs by handing the responsibility of ensuring the safety of their food to the federal government. Consequently, we became separated from our food supply. In 1952, again out of fear, we handed over the responsibility of deciding *what* we should eat. In that year, the government would begin to change the way we *think* about food and, consequently, change our behavior. From that point on, Big Brother would nudge our food choices. And, we would begin to place more trust in the government than in ourselves. In fact, it's happening right now through the seemingly benign *Dietary Guidelines*.

## What Are The Dietary Guidelines?

The *Dietary Guidelines* are a federal document that tells Americans what they should eat, how much they should eat, and which foods they should minimize or avoid.[1] These guidelines are touted by the government as a "critical tool" for medical doctors, dietitians, and nutritionists "to help Americans make healthy choices in their daily lives to help prevent chronic disease and enjoy a healthy diet."[1] That means, the diet advice you receive from a doctor or dietitian most likely adheres to the federal *Dietary Guidelines*.

However, the *primary purpose* of the *Dietary Guidelines* is to develop federal food and health policies and programs. For instance, the *Dietary Guidelines* are used as the foundation in the following federal food programs:

- Both the National School Lunch Program and the School Breakfast Program are built on the *Dietary Guidelines*. Together, these programs feed over 30 million children every school day.
- The Special Supplemental Nutrition Program for Women, Infants, and Children, the "SNAP" welfare program, uses the *Dietary Guidelines* to feed 8 million women, infants, and children every day.
- The Older Americans Act Nutrition Services programs, which is a nutrition program targeting older individuals, feeds over 900,000 people each day based on the *Dietary Guidelines*.[1]

The federal *Dietary Guidelines* also influence what type of research is funded, with our tax dollars, at the National Institute of Health.[2] And, they are used to create educational materials that are disseminated across the country through programs that are designed to teach us how to eat. These programs are used in schools, the Department of Veterans Affairs, the Department of Defense, businesses, the food industry, and even the media. All of the dietary advice that is given to Americans through these programs is required by law to conform to the *Dietary Guidelines*.[1] The *Dietary Guidelines* are also used in grocery stores and on food labels. If you flip over your favorite box of cereal, you'll find "Nutrition Facts" that are based on a 2,000-calorie diet. That's part of the *Dietary Guidelines*. It's a label that is "designed to help you select foods that will meet the *Dietary Guidelines*."[3]

As you can see, the *Dietary Guidelines* are not simply diet recommendations endorsed by our government. They are put into practice in every facet of our lives from schools to hospitals to military bases to grocery stores. If you live in America, you've been affected by these guidelines.

## Brainwashed

Do you remember learning about the food guide pyramid in elementary school? That's part of the *Dietary Guidelines*. That's Big Brother telling you what to eat. They brainwashed us at an early, impressionable age through the public school system. Disagree?

Think about it: The *Dietary Guidelines* **changed our perception of food, which nudges our behavior** in the direction the federal government desires. For instance, when you grab for that fatty cheeseburger, do you hear a voice in the back of your head telling you not to eat it? You know that it's "bad" for you. You know that it's full of fat. But, clearly you want it. Your body might even be craving that cheeseburger. Maybe it wants the fat that's dripping off the sides of the burger. And, why wouldn't it? Fat tastes good, it makes us feel full, it is pleasing to our mouths, and our brains need fat to function properly.[4] So, whose voice is in your head telling you not to eat it?

That's Big Brother.

That's the result of years of brainwashing that began when we were little kids. Here are some additional examples of how the *Dietary Guidelines* might have changed your perception or beliefs about food and, consequently, nudged your behavior:

- If you think eating fat will make you fat.
- If you think low-fat milk is better for you than whole-fat milk.
- If you think you should remove the skin from your chicken before you eat it.
- If you don't remove the skin from your chicken and then you feel bad for eating it.
- Likewise, if you eat the fat on your steak and you feel bad.
- If you think eating red meat is bad for you.
- If you think eating red meat and saturated fat cause heart disease.
- If you think eating lean meat, like skinless chicken and fish, is better for you than eating steak.
- If you think you will live a longer, healthier life by following the *Dietary Guidelines*.
- If you try to avoid saturated fat.
- If you think following the 2,000-calorie diet that is posted on our food labels won't make you fat.

The reason we believe low-fat is good and red meat is bad is because the *Dietary Guidelines* have historically pushed for a low-fat, high-carbohydrate diet.[5] The reason we have an internal debate when we want to eat a fatty cheeseburger or a steak is because of the *Dietary Guidelines*. It was part of the school curriculum when we were children, and it still is today.[6] But, it's even worse today because now the government provides a website for educators so they can be more effective at pushing the *Dietary Guidelines*. The website provides free hand-outs, worksheets, online games, videos, and songs.[7] There is a section on the government website where children can "pledge" to become a "MyPlate Champion." MyPlate is the new Food Guide Pyramid. When I last checked, there were 44,784 children who pledged allegiance to the government to become MyPlate Champions.[6] The brainwashing continues.

Every time you don't listen to your body and, instead, you listen to that voice in your head, you are consenting to Big Brother's authority over your dietary choices. You are allowing the government to nudge your behavior. In addition, you are consenting to wearing the veil: **You are trusting the government to make your food choices, as opposed to trusting yourself.** You are trusting that they know what's best for you and that your own body knows less.

I contend that part of the reason so many of us trust the *Dietary Guidelines* is because the government sold the guidelines to us as fact. They don't present the *Dietary Guidelines* as the best *recommendation* they have at the time based on the available information. Instead, the guidelines are taught as fact: "This is what you should eat. This is what you should not eat." The guidelines are advertised by the federal government as the "solution" and "scientific foundation" that will "help reduce the risk of chronic disease."[1] The government is so confident that they know what's best for us to eat that these guidelines are used to feed millions of people every day, including sick people. They even tell us that these guidelines "can be relied upon to help Americans choose a healthy eating pattern and enjoyable life."[1] There is no humility in these *Dietary Guidelines*. And, there is no humility in the dissemination of the information either.

### What if they're wrong?

What if the federal government has been telling us what to eat for decades, and their advice is actually making us sicker?

## One Man Changes Everything

The *Dietary Guidelines* can be traced back to one man, Ancel Keys. If you recall, we ran into Keys in chapter six. He told us that trans fats were bad, back when the GRAS loophole came into existence. Keys is arguably the most influential man in the history of nutrition. He came up with the idea that eating saturated fat causes heart disease. But his contribution to our culture did not begin and end with a mere hypothesis. Keys managed to convince the American Heart Association (AHA), President Eisenhower, the media, and the public that Americans should eat less saturated fat if they want to avoid heart disease. In doing so, he changed the way that you and I eat today.[8]

Ancel Keys is the man behind the low-fat craze. He's the reason we view fat as "bad." His idea that eating saturated fat causes heart disease developed into the heart-healthy diet that was pushed by the AHA. Do you remember seeing the AHA stamp of approval on certain foods in the grocery store? It's a red heart with a white check that says, "American Heart Association Certified."[9] That stemmed from Ancel Keys' hypothesis. He is also largely responsible for the creation of our *Dietary Guidelines*. Those guidelines recommend that all Americans over the age of 2 cut down on saturated fat, which is another way of saying we should eat less animal meat, dairy, eggs and cheese.[5] And, it all started with this one man and a graph.

In the 1950s, heart disease abruptly showed up on the scene in America.[10] People with no apparent symptoms would suddenly experience a severe pain in their chest and then die. Believe it or not, heart attacks were not common in America before the 1950s. Seemingly overnight, heart disease became the leading cause of death.[8] Understandably, Americans were scared. They wanted answers. What caused this disease? Most importantly, how could they avoid it? One man gave them their answers.

In 1952, Ancel Keys stood in front of a room filled with "experts" and showed them a graph. The message of that graph would change our history: If you don't want to die from heart disease, eat less fat.[11] Suddenly, America had an answer! They didn't have to be afraid of dying any longer. All they had to do was eat less fat and they'd be saved! It might sound crazy that one graph would change the course of our history, but it did. It shaped our entire food system. Disagree?

Do you think that eating too much fat can cause heart disease?

I bet most of us believe that. Why else would we force ourselves to choke down low-fat cookies, low-fat cakes, and skinless chicken breasts? That behavior was set in motion by Ancel Keys. But, he didn't stop at total fat.

By the mid-1950s, Keys no longer blamed total fat for high rates of heart disease. Instead, he isolated a single culprit: saturated fat.[8] Right around the same time, the unexpected happened. President Eisenhower had his first heart attack on September 23, 1955. His medical doctor was named Paul Dudley White. Dr. White had previously spent time with Ancel Keys while traveling to various countries to measure heart disease risks. Consequently, it's no surprise that Dr. White blamed saturated fat for Eisenhower's heart attack. On September 24th, one day after the heart attack, Dr. White held a press conference where he boasted about Ancel Keys while publicly villainizing saturated fat. He lectured Americans on their diet, telling them to avoid saturated fat if they didn't want to have a heart attack.[8] The nation's top doctor had spoken, and America reacted.

The American Heart Association (AHA) formed an expert committee to develop diet advice aimed at preventing heart disease. They initially published a cautious report stating that not enough data existed to make any definitive conclusions about what Americans should and should not eat.[12] Just a few years later, in 1961, the AHA changed course dramatically. They released a second report offering the following advice: If you want to reduce your chance of heart disease, eat less saturated fat.[13] Does that advice sound familiar?

It's Keys' theory.

Ancel Keys and his buddy, Jeremiah Stemler, managed to finagle their way onto the AHA expert committee prior to the release of the second AHA report.[8]

Two weeks after the AHA guidelines were announced, *Time* magazine ran a front-page story praising Ancel Keys and his brilliance.[14] Like clockwork, practitioners began advising their patients to eat a low-fat diet. The media jumped on the bandwagon by promoting the AHA heart-healthy diet in magazine and newspaper articles. People all across the country began to eat less fat and more carbohydrate.[8]

This was a big deal! The AHA recommendation of decreasing saturated fat consumption was the **first official dietary statement ever made by**

**a nationally recognized organization.** Their guideline became the gold standard for diet advice in the United States and around the entire globe.[8]

The only problem is that the recommendations were never validated. **Nobody tested the diet guidelines before they were recommended to the American public.**[8] Nobody fed humans the low-fat diet, based on Keys' theory, and then examined the people to see what happened.

And, remember the graph Keys used in 1952 to convince Americans that fat causes heart disease? Keys hand-selected his data points![8] Data from 22 countries was available at the time, but Keys chose to use data from only six countries. When all of the available data is taken into account, his graph is wrong. Scientists looked at all 22 countries and found that wealth was most strongly correlated with risk of death from heart disease. It wasn't fat. Keys manipulated the data by hand-picking the countries that supported his hypothesis and then publicly pointed the finger at fat.[8] But it gets even worse.

Three years after the AHA guidelines were released, Keys completed a study he believed would support his theory. It's called the Seven Countries study.[15] It was an ambitious undertaking, being the first multi-country epidemiological study in the history of the world. He followed thousands of middle-aged men from the United States, Italy, Greece, Yugoslavia, Finland, Japan, and the Netherlands. He compared their diets with known risks for heart disease. Ancel Keys claimed that this study proved his theory was correct: The more saturated fat you eat, the greater your risk of dying from heart disease.[15] Unfortunately, the study had major flaws:

1.   Have you heard of the Mediterranean diet? It's touted as the diet for Americans to strive for. People from that region reportedly had less heart disease because they ate a diet higher in vegetable fats and lower in animal fats. That conclusion came from Keys' Seven Countries study, and it's flawed.

    Keys sampled the diets of people living in Crete and Corfu three different times. One of the samples was collected during Lent, which means a portion of the study population would have stopped eating animal products, including butter, eggs, and cheese. In fact, the director of the study confirmed that 60% of the study participants were fasting for Lent during the time of the data collection.[16] Why is that a problem?

    It's estimated that saturated-fat intake is cut in half during Lent in Crete.[17] Keys acknowledged the mistake, but dismissed it.

Instead, Keys used the data from that time period to calculate the total amount of saturated fat in the diet of men from Crete, i.e. the Mediterranean diet. He made an error. Consequently, his diet advice to Americans is simply wrong because, outside of Lent, the people of Greece ate more saturated fat than he reported.[18]

2. Keys used three different methods for measuring the amount of fat in the samples of food that he collected. He reported that the results of the three methods were different and he didn't know which data set was accurate.[18]

3. Keys hand-selected countries that he thought would support his theory, just as he did when he previously created the graph that captivated America.[8]

Despite the flaws, the scientific community embraced Keys' Seven Countries study. The AHA published it in 1970. Five books and over 500 articles followed.[15] In addition, it has been referenced by the scientific community an estimated 1 million times.[8] The Seven Countries study became the foundational evidence used to support the dietary advice that Americans have been given for over 50 years: Eat less saturated fat.[8] To this day, our government guidelines still recommend a diet low in fat, including limiting saturated fat intake.[5]

In 1999, almost thirty years after Keys' Seven Countries study was published, the lead Italian researcher in that study re-evaluated the data. He found that sugar was highly correlated with deaths from heart disease. **Sugar was the most likely culprit, not saturated fat.**[19] That's bad news for us because the low-fat foods we've been choking down for decades are typically high in sugar! Fat brings flavor to foods. Consequently, when manufacturers remove fat from our foods, they add sugar to make them taste good again.[20]

Keys, of course, long opposed the sugar hypothesis because if it were true then his saturated fat theory was wrong. He went to great lengths to silence his critics, including publicly discrediting them and even resorting to bullying. If you opposed his saturated fat theory, you were at risk of losing your funding, your job, your ability to publish your work in reputable journals, and even speaking engagements.[8]

To this day:

• Research has not conclusively shown that eating saturated fat causes the damaging type of cholesterol to increase.[21]

- Research has not conclusively shown that elevated total cholesterol means you have an increased risk of developing a heart attack.[21]
- Research has not conclusively shown that if your arteries narrow you are more likely to have a heart attack.[8]

Yet, the AHA still pushes Keys' saturated fat theory by recommending we all reduce our saturated fat, including eating less meat and whole-fat dairy.[22†] People follow this advice because the AHA remains our leading "expert" in heart disease prevention. That fascinates me because Cocoa Puffs used to carry the trusted AHA heart-check seal of

## SEASONING

### "Experts" Encouraged Americans to Eat Tran Fats

Procter & Gamble gave Crisco® to America in 1911, which was the first hydrogenated oil in our diets.[23] The AHA endorsed Crisco®. In fact, the medical director of the AHA posed on camera with a bottle of Crisco®. The AHA was a small group with no money until Procter & Gamble gave them $17 million (in today's money), which may have influenced that endorsement.[8] Regardless, AHA "experts" ensured the American people that Crisco®, and other hydrogenated oils that came from vegetables, were safe and healthy. They encouraged Americans to eat them as a replacement for animal fat. Americans complied. We switched from eating animal fats and no vegetable oils before 1910, to consuming roughly 8% of our total calories from vegetable oils by 1999.[24] So, what's the problem?

The rise in consumption of vegetable oils matches perfectly with the rise in heart disease that plagued Americans during the mid-1900s.[8] It might be a coincidence, but it's certainly worth pondering. It's also noteworthy that Crisco® contains trans fats, which are now essentially banned from the market because of their direct link to heart disease.[25] Yet, at the time, the leading "experts" in heart disease (i.e., the AHA) advised Americans to eat Crisco® if they wanted to avoid heart disease.

---

† For an in-depth look into how nutrition science got the Dietary Guidelines wrong, I recommend reading *The Big Fat Surprise* by investigative journalist Nina Teicholz.

approval. That doesn't sound like a heart healthy food to me, but what do I know? I'm also just an "expert" in food.

## Government Grabs Hold Of Our Cheeseburgers

After the AHA dietary guidelines were released and implemented, disease rates continued to increase in America.[26,27] Consequently, the government got serious about "helping" Americans live healthier and more "enjoyable" lives.[5] **In 1977, the federal government became an active participant in our daily food choices.** It started with one government report, which would become the most influential document in the history of diet and disease.[28] The Senate Select Committee on Nutrition and Human Needs released a report called *Dietary Goals for the United States*. That report contained the first official U.S. government dietary recommendations.[29] Can you guess what diet advice the Senate committee provided to Americans?

Eat less saturated fat.[29]

The Senate committee was comprised of former journalists and lawyers. Nobody was a doctor or nutritionist.[29] Nobody had medical or dietary expertise. What the committee did have was politics and bias:

- Senator George McGovern led the Senate Committee. Just prior to the committee hearings, Senator McGovern participated in a weeklong clinic based on the low-fat diet teachings of Nathan Pritikin, a famous diet guru. Clearly, McGovern was biased.
- Nick Mottern was the staffer in charge of conducting research for the group, as well as writing the report. He was a progressive who fought against the big, bad corporations, particularly the meat, dairy and egg industries. Prior to working on the Senate committee, Mottern reported on unfair labor practices for a small newspaper. Since Mottern had essentially no knowledge of nutrition, he relied on Dr. Mark Hegsted.
- Dr. Hegsted was a professor of Nutrition at the Harvard School of Public Health. Dr. Hegsted was also a staunch supporter of Keys' saturated fat hypothesis.[8]

Consequently, it's no surprise that the Senate report concluded: Americans should eat a diet low in fat, especially saturated fat. In lock step with the AHA, the *Dietary Goals* consisted of the following recommendations:

- Reduce overall fat intake from 40% of your daily calories to 30%.
- Eat no more saturated fat than 10% of your daily calories.
- Increase carbohydrate intake to 55-60% of your daily calories.[29]

Does that sound familiar?

Those recommendations are still the basis of our *Dietary Guidelines* today.[5]

Mottern was likely thrilled with these guidelines since the meat, dairy, and egg industries got snubbed.[8] Recommending Americans eat less saturated fat translated into eating less animal products, including meat, dairy, and eggs. How do you think those industries responded to the newly announced *Dietary Goals*?

They sent lobbyists straight to Senator McGovern's office to have a little chat. Suffice it to say, an exception for lean meat was carved out.[8] That's why the government tells us it's okay to eat fish and chicken, as long as you remove the skin, but it's not okay to eat red meat, butter, eggs, and whole milk products like full-fat yogurt.[8]

Meanwhile, the large food manufacturers were thrilled. Advising Americans to eat more carbohydrate benefitted the cereal and grain companies like Quaker Oats® and General Foods®. Interestingly, these companies had already developed a cozy relationship with academia by supplying them with money to fund scientific research and hosting influential conferences. With their hand directly in the cookie jar, the food industry was able to sway the opinions of researchers, government officials, and the public.[8] Is it possible that the food industry influenced the outcome of the *Dietary Goals* in 1977?

Common sense tells us yes.

For better or worse, America was handed a set of *Dietary Goals* that were created largely by one man, based on a false narrative, likely influenced by industry, and never properly reviewed or tested.[8]

**Those *Dietary Goals* became the *rules* that Americans are supposed to follow and that all government food policies are based upon.**

## Americans Should Eat 13 Slices Of Bread Each Day

Dr. Mark Hegsted, who Mottern enlisted to be the brains behind the *Dietary Goals*, became the chief administrator of those recommendations. He was in charge of translating the guidelines into practice. By 1978, the best the USDA could come up with was a recommendation for Americans to eat 13 slices of bread to meet their daily carbohydrate needs.[30]

## America Consents

The 1977 *Dietary Goals for the United States* evolved into the *Dietary Guidelines for Americans* that we know today. As of 1990, the federal government is *required by law* to release a new set of *Dietary Guidelines* every five years. Specifically, the National Nutrition Monitoring and Related Research Act requires the USDA and the Department of Health and Human Services to publish a report, every five years, telling Americans what they should and shouldn't eat.[31] It's absurd that a federal law was passed requiring our government to tell us how we should eat, including which foods are "bad" and which are "good," and how much of each food we should be allowed to eat. Clearly, the government thinks it knows best when it comes to the foods we put in our bodies.

Yet, the mere fact that the guidelines are updated every 5 years implies that the government doesn't have the answer. If the *Dietary Guidelines* were truly the answer that would "solve" the issue of chronic illness that America is facing, as they claim it is, surely the answer would not have to be revised every 5 years.[1] I give the federal government credit for acknowledging that the state of the science can change, so the guidelines may need to be updated accordingly. However, they present the guidelines as *the* solution rather than a recommendation. As previously noted, these guidelines have an unprecedented influence on Americans. They set policies that reach into our schools, hospitals, veterans' facilities, and every federal agency imaginable. Shouldn't we be absolutely certain that the "solution" is correct before unleashing it into every nook and cranny of our lives?

Regardless, Americans have bought into this system. We have acquiesced authority over our food choices. We have stopped listening to our bodies and our intuition. Our inner voice has been replaced by the dictatorial voice of Big Brother telling us, "That's bad for you. Don't eat that." Even the AHA encourages us to hand authority of our food choices to them with their current slogan: "Let our heart be your guide."[32] In other words, "Don't rely on your own heart, or intuition, to guide your decision, trust our heart instead." And, people do! As a child, I remember watching my Mother look for the AHA heart-check of approval. We bought into the system. We consented. But, who's advice have we consented to? Who creates the *Dietary Guidelines*?

A group of 11-15 "experts" on the Dietary Guidelines Advisory Committee advise both the USDA and HHS on what Americans should eat. The recommendations of that group become the *Dietary Guidelines*. According to a 2015 report in the *British Medical Journal*:

> "The scientific committee advising the US government…relies heavily on systematic reviews from professional bodies such as the American Heart Association and the American College of Cardiology, which are heavily supported by food and drug companies."[2]

In other words, **the food and drug industries have largely determined the dietary rules that all Americans should follow**. And, we've consented.

So, what has our consent gotten us?

## Sicker America

We have dutifully changed our eating habits. In the 1800s we ate much more meat than we do today, and it was predominantly red meat. For instance, we likely ate 175 pounds of meat per person each year in the 1800s.[33] Today, we eat roughly 100 pounds of meat per person each year and roughly half of that meat is in the form of lean meats, including chicken and turkey.[34] We also ate a lot more butter than we do now. Today we eat less than four pounds per person each year. In the 1800s, we ate roughly 16 pounds of butter per person each year![35] Clearly we've changed our diets, shifting away from red meat and saturated fats. So, are we all leading "healthier" and more "enjoyable" lives, like the federal government promised we would be if we just followed their *Dietary Guidelines*?

No. Actually, we're sicker.

By the government's own admission, half of us currently have at least one chronic disease, including: diabetes, heart disease, obesity, and cancer.[1] In addition, we are more obese than ever. When the AHA recommended we eat their heart-healthy diet, roughly one in seven adults were obese.[26] That number climbed to more than one in three adults just 50 years later.[36] Obesity has become such a national crisis that the federal government launched a program called "Healthy People" with the goal of lowering the obesity level to what we had in the 1960s, just before the *Dietary Guidelines* were introduced.[1,8] And, what happened to our risk for heart disease? It's the reason we got into this mess in the first place. Has our risk dropped since the government swooped in to "solve" the problem?

Nope.

Heart disease is still the leading cause of death in America.[37]

Can someone please remind me why we need the government to teach us how to eat?

## Losing Our Freedom

Not only are Americans sicker today after following the governments' dietary recommendations, we are less free. By allowing the government to dictate what we should eat and how much, **we have consented to Big Brother removing our freedom of choice**. We have set the stage to allow the federal government to remove personal choice and replace it with a dictatorship. What if the government decides it has the authority to ban foods that it declares to be unhealthy, like our juicy cheeseburger? If that sounds too far-fetched, look no further than the 18th Amendment.

In 1919, the federal government banned alcohol at the national level. Think about that for a moment: Our government passed a *constitutional amendment* that made it illegal for us to consume a particular food. Why would we ever give a government that authority? Today they might ban alcohol and you might be okay with that. But, what if tomorrow our government decided to ban your large soda? Too late!

The former mayor Michael Bloomberg already tried that in New York City. Luckily, it was rejected by the state's highest court, citing that the government had "exceeded the scope of its regulatory authority."[38]

Banning food hasn't been wildly successful in America, but taxing food is gaining momentum. For example, in June of 2016, the Philadelphia City Council approved a 1.5-cent-per-ounce tax on soda, which is projected to increase the cost of a two-liter bottle of soda by roughly $1.00.[39] In a 13-4 vote, a government council ushered in the first-ever government-imposed soda tax under the guise that it will reduce obesity and help lift people out of poverty.[39] The tax may accomplish those goals, but at what cost?

Each time we allow government to influence our behavior, in this case by targeting our food, we lose more of our liberty. Taxing food may initially seem like a good idea. It could lead to a healthier America by lowering the obesity rate. And, it sounds better than the government banning food. At least you still have a choice, right?

Actually, taxing food is arguably worse than banning food because it's sneaky. Instead of outlawing a food, which could cause uproar by consumers, the government slowly nudges us away from a particular food by providing market incentives, or disincentives in this case. For instance, by increasing the cost of soda, government nudges us away from it. Once the tax is in place, most likely at some low, barely noticeable level, government can slowly raise the tax level to nudge your behavior further. Eventually, you can't afford the soda any longer. But, at least you still have a choice, right? There's even a name for this strategy: libertarian paternalism. The bottom line is: Taxing food drives us further from a free market and closer to serfdom.

But, some people don't see it that way. Or, maybe they are unaware of what's at stake because *the people* are voting to impose food taxes on themselves. For example:

- In 2014, voters in Berkeley, California, approved the first tax on soda at the local level.[40]
- In November of 2016, voters in Boulder, Colorado and three cities in California (San Francisco, Albany, and Oakland) approved a tax on sugar-sweetened beverages, like soda.[41]

I wouldn't be surprised if a soda tax becomes federal law in the near future. After all, in 2015, the Dietary Guidelines Advisory Committee recommended the federal government impose a tax on soda and sugary snacks.[40] And, President Obama's former chief economic advisor, Larry Summers, declared, "Mark my words, this one will come."[42]

In addition, now that the Affordable Care Act is in play, what's stopping the government from penalizing you for behaviors they feel are unhealthy or costly to the system? If you are overweight or obese, you are more likely to rack up higher health care costs. Why should the government, by way of the taxpayers, pick up your tab? Perhaps the government will decide to increase premiums for anyone who is overweight. We've already heard President Barack Obama say to the American people that it's not *fair* he has to pay the health care costs of someone who abuses their body.[28]

My point is: When will it stop? Where will the line be drawn? Who decides what is "good" for you and what is "bad" for you to eat? Clearly, if that decision is left to the government then we're all in trouble.

## You Hold The Answer

As an "expert" in Nutrition, I am not advising Americans to eat more red meat or saturated fat. That's an individual choice that you can decide for yourself. And I'm not suggesting that all of the *Dietary Guidelines* are bad. Clearly, you're better off not eating doughnuts and chocolate milk for breakfast. But, do we really need Big Brother to tell us that?

When it comes to our daily food choices, a consequence of giving our consent to Big Brother is that we've lost touch with our own bodies. If you pay attention to how your body responds to foods you choose to eat, it will tell you what it wants and what it doesn't want.[‡] If you choose to eat a breakfast of doughnuts and chocolate milk, you will enjoy a sugar high followed by an unpleasant sugar crash. You may feel tired, unmotivated, cranky, and have a bad craving for more sugar. That sugar crash is your body's way of telling you to "knock it off." Or, let's say you love spicy food, but every time you eat it you get heartburn. That's your body saying, "Please don't eat that." What about that fat, juicy cheeseburger we talked about? If your body is craving that burger, then it's clearly telling you it needs the nutrients in that food. Maybe it needs the fat, or perhaps it wants the iron?

---

‡ For information on how to reconnect with your body, please refer to *BodyWise* by Dr. Rachel Abrams.

HANDS OFF MY FOOD!

My point is that we are individuals. Our response to the foods we eat depends on many factors including: ancestry, genetics, nutritional status, stress level, age, gender, and emotional state. Consequently, the one size fits all government approach to our *Dietary Guidelines* doesn't work. It's like a shirt that is labeled as one size fits all. It's a good idea, but in reality it hardly fits anyone. The same holds true for *Dietary Guidelines*. You cannot "guide" an *individual* to health and wellness by prescribing *generalized* guidelines. Years ago, I attended a scientific conference in Boston where a researcher presented startling findings from a study he had just conducted. He fed people omega-3 fatty acid supplements and then measured the triglyceride level in their blood. He expected everyone's triglycerides to decrease. That's not what happened. Roughly one-third of the people did experience a decrease, but one-third showed no change in triglycerides and the remaining one-third of people showed an increase! Confusing, right? That's why generalized recommendations don't work. We are individuals.

Only you can decide which foods are "good" for you and which foods are "bad." Nobody knows your body better than you do. **As long as you can differentiate between what your body needs and what your mind craves, you are the best dietitian or nutritionist that money can buy.** But, many of us have lost the ability to understand our bodies. The connection between our mind, body, and spirit has been severed. Consequently, when determining our own dietary needs, we've lost trust in ourselves. We began to lose that trust the day we put more faith in Big Brother than ourselves; the day we replaced our intuition, our inner voice, with the voice of Big Brother. Consequently, we are more removed from our food and from ourselves than ever before in American history.

## What You Can Do

- **Listen to your body:** Learn to distinguish between what your body needs and what your mind wants.
- **Reconnect with your food** by practicing mindful eating:
  - Instead of eating while distracted (i.e. watching TV, working, or reading), sit down at a table and focus on your food. Taste each bite. Take note of the flavors, colors, smells, and textures.

o Before you eat, express gratitude for your food through prayer, meditation, or positive thoughts.
o Chew each bite 30 times. Notice how the taste and texture of the food changes as you continue to chew.
- **Support the Nutrition Coalition:** I do not support federal dietary guidelines. However, in the absence of eliminating the program entirely, the next best option is to support organizations that are working to strengthen the guidelines by ensuring they are based on accurate and conclusive science. The Nutrition Coalition is a nonprofit advocacy organization working to achieve accurate guidelines by basing recommendations on sound science and getting rid of the one-size fits all approach. (www.nutrition-coalition.org)

## Take Home Message

The *Dietary Guidelines* began out of fear. Americans were dying from heart disease and they wanted answers. They got them in the form of a biased, flawed, and untested hypothesis that remains the basis of our *Dietary Guidelines* today. Those guidelines dictate federal food and health policy, but they also nudge our behavior. The *Dietary Guidelines* have fundamentally changed the way we view food. In the end, our consent has made us sicker and has jeopardized our freedom. By placing more trust in the government than ourselves, we have become further separated from our food. Even worse, we have become separated from ourselves.

## Moving Forward

Are you ready to do something about our food supply? Are you fed up with being an un-consenting guinea pig? Are you tired of eating plastic in your cupcakes? Are you concerned about feeding your children GMOs? If you answered yes to any of these questions then join me for section three of this book where we discuss how to restore our food supply, *one small step at a time.*

# SECTION 3:

# EASY WAYS TO FIGHT BACK

# CHAPTER 10

# POWER OF THE PEOPLE

The lack of integrity in our food supply is real and it affects all of us because we all eat food. Now that your veil of unearned trust in our food supply has hopefully been lifted, what will you do with this knowledge? Will you fight to change it? Or, will you continue with your normal daily routine, knowing there is a problem but thinking it's too big for any one person to make a difference?

I can't tell you how many times I've heard someone say, "I'm just one person, what difference can I make?" Or, "I'm one person, my vote won't make a difference." That disposition means we've been conditioned to give up before we even begin to fight. I refuse to resign myself to that state of lackadaisical defeat. I realize that fighting for our food supply is a full-blown case of David and Goliath. I'm not in denial. The odds are against us. Protecting our food supply means fighting against government, industry, "experts," and lobbyists backed by deep pockets. Fortunately for us, we have a model to learn from.

The odds were stacked against us when we fought for our Independence. The British were the most powerful military force in the world at that time. America didn't even have a military. Our soldiers were farmers and shopkeepers who were not trained for combat. In addition, only a minority of Americans supported the Revolution. It's estimated that roughly one-third of the colonists wanted independence, one-third wanted to remain ruled by a king, and one-third were silent or didn't want to be involved.[1] In other words, America exists today because of a minority of individuals who chose freedom over slavery and silence.

How did a minority of farmers and shopkeepers win a war against the greatest military force in the world?

Dedication to the cause and commitment to each other were the keys to victory. The one-third of Americans that fought for our freedom pledged their "lives, fortunes, and sacred honor." Their commitment ran so deep that they publicly declared they would die just so you and I could be free. They stood side by side through seemingly insurmountable odds, knowing that if they were captured they could be killed for treason. It took seven years, but they eventually did win freedom for "ourselves and our posterity."

It's astounding what a minority of individuals can do when they are committed. It reminds me of the words of Margaret Mead, the cultural anthropologist who helped spark the feminist movement:

"Never doubt that a small group of thoughtful, committed citizens can change the word; indeed, it's the only thing that ever has."[2]

History tells us that **"a small group" can change the world**. We saw this happen with the birth of America as well as with the birth of Israel. I was taught that Moses led *all* of the Jews out of Egypt during the Exodus. That may not actually be true. According to rabbinic scholar Rabbi Daniel Lapin, roughly 20% of enslaved Jews left with Moses.[3†] The rest stayed behind. That means roughly 80% of Jews chose slavery over freedom. Only a minority of Jews left bondage to seek out the promise land. I find that fascinating. If I had a choice, I'd like to think I'd choose freedom every time. But, history tells us that not everyone chooses freedom because freedom isn't free. Freedom comes at a price. Consequently, some choose to be ruled by a king or pharaoh. They choose to remain trapped in the system.

Which will you choose?

---

† According to Rabbi Lapin, "20% of Israelites are recorded as having left Egypt. The relevant verse is Exodus 13:18. Most English translations mistakenly translate it as Children of Israel went up from Egypt "armed". The King James used "harnessed". The Hebrew says "Chamushim" meaning 1/5. (The Hebrew word for five is CHaMeSH) There is nowhere else in Scripture that translators claim this word means 'armed'."

Will you choose to remain enslaved by our food supply; a system that is corrupted by money and backdoor deals and is controlled by a handful of influential individuals? Will you be part of the group that remains silent? Or, will you fight to restore the integrity of the very food that you and your children eat every day?

## The Power Of One

If we ban together, all we need is a minority to change the entire system, but it starts with the individual. It starts with each one of us. If you don't think one person can change the system, I'd like you to meet Sarah Kavanagh.

When she was just 15-years old, Sarah Kavanagh launched an online campaign against Gatorade®. Sarah loved drinking Gatorade®. But, one day, she read the ingredient label on the back of the bottle. One ingredient in particular, brominated vegetable oil (BVO), seemed disturbing. So, she began doing her own research.

Sarah learned that BVO is a flame retardant. She also learned that it was banned in Gatorade® sold in Europe and Japan, but it was allowed in Gatorade® sold in the U.S. Why the discrepancy between the U.S. and other countries?

Sarah didn't want to give up drinking her Gatorade®, but she also didn't want to drink BVO. So, she started an online petition against PepsiCo Inc., the maker of Gatorade®. In her petition, Sarah wrote:

> "According to Scientific America…It [BVO] is 'under intense scrutiny because research has shown that they are building up in people's bodies, including breast milk, around the world.' The same article also mentions that there are 'links to impaired neurological development, reduced fertility, early onset of puberty and altered thyroid hormones.'" [4]

It took two years, but Sarah won her fight! PepsiCo Inc. removed BVO from its products. They released a statement acknowledging the removal was due to consumer pushback. In that statement, PepsiCo Inc. also affirmed that they did nothing wrong because the FDA allows this chemical to be used in food products:

> "While our products are safe, we are making this change because we know that some consumers have a negative perception of

BVO in Gatorade, despite being permitted for use in North American and Latin American countries."[5]

In lock step, the FDA came to the defense of PepsiCo Inc., claiming BVO is safe for us to drink:

"Based on several long-term animal studies…the FDA has determined that BVO is safe and presents no health risks."[5]

Not surprisingly, BVO is derived from corn and soy, which are probably subsidized and genetically modified. In addition, BVO was designated as GRAS in 1958. Remember our old friend GRAS? It's the loophole that allows industry to decide which chemicals are safe for us to eat without any oversight by the FDA. Well, after making the GRAS list by default, in the 1970s the FDA stripped BVO of GRAS status based on concerns of possible heart issues related to BVO consumption. The FDA decided BVO could still be used as a food additive "on an interim basis…pending the outcome of additional toxicological studies…"[6,7] We're still waiting on the outcome of the studies. Meanwhile, BVO is still found in roughly 10% of sodas in the U.S. along with some sports drinks, energy drinks, and fruit drinks.[8,9]

Let's take a moment to reflect on this situation: A 15-year old girl stood up against PepsiCo Inc., a $127 billion company, and she won. Talk about David and Goliath! Incredibly, it all began with a teenager reading a food label. So, how did she defeat Goliath?

Sarah was able to rally enough people to support her cause by launching an online campaign with a common sense, simple message: "Don't put flame retardant chemicals in sports drinks!"[4] It only took a minority of Americans to engage in the fight before PepsiCo Inc. succumbed to consumer pressure. Just over 200,000 people signed her online petition. That's roughly 0.067% of our population. That's all it took!

Sarah's story is proof that we don't need to move mountains to change our food supply. We simply need to move one shovel full of dirt at a time. If we all carry just one shovel of dirt, we can build a *new* mountain. In other words, we can change our food supply by taking back our consent.

## Consent

Whether you realize it or not, you impact our food supply every time you eat. The market moves based on how you spend your money, which means you are exerting your power every day through the food choices you make. It also means you are giving your consent based on how you spend your money. Every time you buy food from a grocery store, restaurant, fast food chain, or vending machine, you financially support those companies. If those companies stand for principles that you are against, you just added to their bottom line instead of being true to yourself. You consented to the principles of that company. In other words, you sacrificed your principles to support theirs.

On the other hand, you can choose to stay true to your principles by giving your consent to companies that are aligned with your values and principles. You have a choice! That's the beauty of the free market. With every food choice you make throughout the day, you can choose to either support the current system or change it. You get to decide if you want to help restore the integrity of our food supply or be complicit in its demise.

*Gut check:* **What are you saying with your dollars?** Are you contributing to the problem or are you helping your cause?

Perhaps you are not currently making conscious decisions in the marketplace based on your values and principles. Perhaps you've never thought of it that way before. I never did. I used to make decisions based on cost, fat content, sodium level, and appearance. Then, one day, I realized that I was giving my consent. I was giving it in an uneducated and haphazard manner, but I was sill consenting:

- I was giving my consent to eating foods that were fundamentally transformed from how God created them.
- I was giving my consent to having steroids pumped into my milk.
- I was giving my consent for the government to hire Monsanto employees that approved the very same research that they conducted when they worked at Monsanto.
- I was giving my consent to be a guinea pig for our government and the food industry.

It doesn't matter that I was unaware of my actions. I was still consenting. I was *silently* giving my consent.

"Silence in the face of evil is itself evil: God will not hold us guiltless. Not to speak is to speak. Not to act is to act."

Dietrich Bonhoeffer spoke those immortal words. He was a Protestant minister who stood up for the Jews during Hitler's reign. He was killed in a concentration camp for speaking out against evil. Unlike so many who chose to remain silent, Bonhoeffer made a decision to speak.

Bonhoeffer knew that silence is a choice.

When you are silent, you are choosing to be complicit in the act. Many of us have been silent in the demise of our food supply, including me. I have spent most of my life in silence. Our silence does not exempt us from the problem. It doesn't give us a free pass. It just makes us part of the problem.

## Who Holds The Power?

Sarah's online campaign against PepsiCo Inc. is a perfect example of how the consumer can change our food supply. It reminds us that **the power lies within the people.** Did you know that? Did you know that our Republic was built on the premise that all power lies within the people? It's written in the Declaration of Independence:

> "We hold these truths to be self-evident, that all men are created equal, that they are endowed by their Creator with certain unalienable Rights, that among these are Life, Liberty and the pursuit of Happiness.—That to secure these rights, Governments are instituted among Men, *deriving their just powers from the consent of the governed...*"[10] [emphasis added]

The power comes from the "consent of the governed." In other words, the power comes from the people and government is only as "powerful" as we, the people, allow it to be.

Let's think about that for just a moment: Arguably, the most "powerful" man in the world is the U.S. President. What would happen if nobody showed up to the polls to re-elect the President of the United States? He'd be fired. Why? He didn't have the support of the people. Some people would say that he lost his "power" because he lost the White House. In reality, he did not lose power because he never had our power to begin with. He lost his authority over the people because we, the people, took back our consent. In other words, he lost "the consent of the governed."

In 2015, I attended an invitation-only roundtable discussion with my Congressman. He invited the heads of political organizations from our district. The moderator, who was an elected party official, started the meeting by emphatically telling all of us how "lucky" we were to be there. In a rather condescending voice, he said we were all "fortunate to be in their presence." As I looked around the room to gauge the reaction of the roughly 35 people in attendance, nearly every person was nodding their head in agreement. One person even said "Thank you" out loud as the moderator was droning on about how "privileged" we all were to be "in the same room" with those select political leaders. This continued for several minutes. As the others were nodding their heads like trained government servants, I thought to myself, "How 'powerful' would you be if all 35 of us got up from this table and walked out of the room?" In other words, how much authority would he have if he lost the consent of the governed? He's only as "powerful" as the people who are supporting him. I'm ashamed to say that I previously supported him. I was one of the delegates who voted him into his position. I consented to his elitist attitude with my vote. Never again would I make that mistake. I pledged to myself, in that moment, to exercise my power by not voting for him again.

"We the people" hold the reins of power over our government, and our power works the same way in the marketplace. Companies are only as "powerful" as we, the consumers, allow them to be. Admittedly, it is complicated because many companies are in bed with the government. But the principle is the same: The government and industry are only as "powerful" as the people allow them to be. I commonly hear people say, "We need to take back Washington." Or, "We need to take back our power." The truth is that we don't need to "take back" our power because we never lost it. The power lies within us.

Once you understand that "we the people" have the power, the next step is to understand where that power comes from. According to the Declaration of Independence, that power is given to us by the "Laws of Nature and of Nature's God."

> "When in the Course of human events, it becomes necessary for one people to dissolve the political bands which have connected them with another, and to assume among the powers of the earth, the separate and equal station to which the *Laws*

*of Nature and of Nature's God entitle them,* a decent respect to the opinions of mankind requires that they should declare the causes which impel them to the separation." [emphasis added]

A higher being gave us our power. That higher being can be whatever you want it to be, as long as it's not human. For example, it can be "Nature's God," or Mother Earth, or Nature, or the Spiritual World, etc. According to the Founders, the higher being was our "Creator" or God.

The important point to remember is that our power does not come from man. That means **no man can take away your power.** No government can take your power from you unless, of course, they kill you. Additionally, you cannot give your power to the government or to industry.

You can give your consent to the government. And, you can give your consent to industry. **Our consent is what gives them authority and influence over our food supply.** But, you cannot give them your power. Therefore, to change our food supply, you simply need to **selectively give your consent.** That is how you effectively assert your power.

## Take Home Message

Power lies within the people. You exercise your power through your consent. What are you saying with your dollars?

## Moving Forward

Now that we know who holds the power, let's learn how to selectively give our consent by 'feeding the good and starving the bad.'

## CHAPTER 11

# FEED THE GOOD, STARVE THE BAD

I used to make phone calls and send emails to companies asking for ingredient changes and sharing scientific research to support my requests. I still use these approaches at times. However, I've learned a more effective method. I speak with my dollars.

Whether you agree with it or not, our food supply boils down to the dollar. That's what shifts the market. That's what keeps companies accountable. Fortunately, as consumers, we largely determine a company's profits. Have you ever thought about that? *We* determine a company's profit. If we don't buy what a company is selling, they lose money. If we do buy what they sell, the company prospers. That's good news for us because it means each of us has the ability to change our food supply by changing the profits of companies.

My main strategy for restoring the integrity of our food supply centers on 'feeding the good and starving the bad.' I exercise my consent by starving the companies I disagree with and feeding the companies that support my cause and my values. I do this in baby steps, changing one food purchase at a time. After all, it took years to arrive at our current diet. It's going to take time to reverse it. So, I recommend picking one goal to focus on at a time. Since GMOs are my big issue, the first change I made in my family's food supply was to only buy non-GMO foods.

The single task of avoiding GMOs quickly became overwhelming for me. I spent hours in the grocery store reading every food label as I tried to figure out which products contained GMOs. Who has time for that? Then I learned that a company can claim their product is non-GMO even if it isn't. Who's regulating that label?

Additionally, I knew that roughly 75% of all processed foods contain GMOs.[1] Hence, for me, it became easier to assume that all processed foods contain at least one genetically modified ingredient unless the package contains the Butterfly.

## Look For The Butterfly

The Butterfly is the seal of the Non-GMO Project. As previously mentioned, the Non-GMO Project is a non-profit, independent organization dedicated to preserving and building the non-GMO food supply. They provide verified non-GMO choices that are easy to spot in the grocery store because their seal of approval is a colorful butterfly that is usually printed on the front of food products. The Butterfly is the most trusted label available for GMO avoidance.[†]

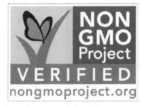

*Figure 1.* Look for the Non-GMO Project Verified butterfly seal when seeking trusted non-GMO products.

Even as a 5-year old, my son could recognize the Butterfly almost immediately when we walked down the processed food aisles. He knew that we only purchased processed foods if they contained that independent verification label. It was always rewarding to see him walk through the grocery store aisles and pick out his own food with purpose and understanding. For instance, when he picked out a container of cookies that had the Butterfly label, he would often shout with excitement, "Look, Mom! Butterfly! No GMOs. Let's buy these!"

Children are smart. I find that they often don't get the credit they deserve. And, if we teach them where their food comes from, they are more likely to make good choices on their own, both now and in the future. For example, when I explained how GM crops are made and how they differ from non-GM crops, my son thought for a moment and

---

† Due to the high risk of contamination, the claim "GMO free" is not legally or scientifically defensible. The Non-GMO Project Standard follows best practices for meaningful GMO avoidance and includes third-party testing, traceability and segregation.

then said to me, "I don't want to eat GMOs. That's not God's food. I want to eat the food God gave us." I could not have said it better myself.

Looking for the Butterfly is a perfect strategy for me because it's a small-government approach that utilizes the free market and maximizes personal responsibility. The government can make mistakes with seemingly no consequences, but an independent company has an incentive to stay on high ground. Unlike the government, if the Non-GMO Project makes a mistake, they could go out of business. Besides, why would we rely on government mandated labeling?

Loopholes always appear, just as we saw with the DARK Act. In addition, mandated labeling provides a false sense of security, which only grows our veils. Therefore, supporting the Non-GMO Project is my way of 'feeding the good and starving the bad.' It is a limited-government approach to the labeling issue, which I can feel good about because it fits with my core principles.

When I buy products that are non-GMO verified, I not only support the companies that are aligned with my passion and principles, I starve the companies that support GMOs. Taking away profits sends a loud and clear message to a company. And, it works. According to A.C. Gallo, President of Whole Foods, once an existing product earns the Butterfly seal, sales soar 15-30%.[2] If we work together, companies that currently supply us with GMO foods will decide that it's in their best interest to stop. They will remove GMOs from our foods once we refuse to buy their products.

If GMOs are not your passion, check out www.handsoffmyfood. com for a free guide containing additional ideas on how to move the market in other areas of our food supply.

## Support Third Party Watchdogs

Whenever possible, I support third party watchdogs. The Non-GMO Project and the Environmental Working Group (EWG) are two watchdogs that I currently support. We've discussed the Non-GMO Project already. For more information, including free access to their product database, visit them at: www.NonGMOProject.org

The goal of the EWG is to help you find products that are safe for us, as well as the environment. They conduct tests on our food, personal care products, and cleaning supplies. Then, they report the results in free guides that are posted on their website. The guides are designed to help you make informed choices, including: which fruits have less pesticides, which sunscreens are the least toxic, and even which cosmetics are the least harmful to your body. Visit www.ewg.org for the free guides.

## Eating Out

Consumer pressure is also moving the fast food marketplace. McDonald's® announced in 2015 that they are changing their policy based on customer demand.[3] McDonald's® customers wanted chicken without antibiotics and McDonald's® responded to that pressure. They promised that within two years, they would only sell chicken that has not been given antibiotics that are used in human medicine. A year before McDonald's® announcement, Chick-fil-A® announced a similar five-year plan that would take effect in all of their stores nation-wide. Chick-fil-A® also removed artificial dyes from some of their dipping sauces. Why?

"Consumers are demanding the change."[4]

Some food chains, like Chipotle®, have restricted antibiotic use in their meats for years. However, Chipotle® has recently stepped up to the plate again in two big ways. First, they removed GMOs from their menu. Second, they fired their pork supplier because they were treating animals with cruelty. Chipotle® was so strong in their stance against animal cruelty that they made the business decision to take a short-term hit: They didn't have any pork to sell until they found a new supplier.[5]

Panera® has also recently been on the frontline in terms of making changes to the fast food industry. Part of their food policy includes using less antibiotics and supporting sustainable fishing and farming. In addition, Panera® announced they will remove all artificial additives by 2016. That means Panera® will eliminate all dyes, preservatives, and artificial sweeteners from their menu. According to their chief concept officer, Scott Davis:

> "Panera is on a mission to help fix a broken food system. We have a long journey ahead, but we're working closely with the nutrition community, industry experts, farmers, suppliers, and others to make a difference."[6]

The bottom line is the customer has the most influence on what is served in restaurants. Money talks. Therefore, feed companies that are aligned with you and starve companies that are not. And, if you don't find a place that is in alignment with your passion and core principles, you now have a potential business idea. Maybe you are destined to venture out and start your own business. I love supporting companies that started from a passion and have a family feel. These companies sometimes write their story on their products. For example, I buy the best tasting coconut chips from a company called Dang®. They are non-GMO, gluten-free, and vegan. The product label states:

> "Dang is my Mother's name. One day she gave me a recipe that required toasted coconut. When I made it I was blown away by the fantastic flavor, so I started selling toasted coconut chips at local markets. Everybody loved them, so I started a company and named it Dang as an homage to my Mom."

This is a great marketing strategy because the story gives us an emotional attachment to the company and the product. Some of us are more likely to support a company we feel a connection with. So, if you have a unique idea for our food supply that is screaming to be explored, consider getting out there and connecting with the people. It just might resonate with us. And, it just might change your life.

## Buy From Local Farmers You Trust

Another way I feed the good and starve the bad is to buy local. Many of us are conditioned to only buy our groceries from the supermarket. We may occasionally shop at a farmer's market, but the overwhelming majority of us primarily buy food from large grocery store chains. Recently, I have made an effort to know my local farmers. I don't immediately hand over my trust just because they are local and own small, family farms. Instead, I give them an opportunity to earn my trust. I do this by being a detective.

First, I conduct a casual interview with them by phone. I ask questions such as:

- What prescription drugs do you give the animals?
- Are they free to graze on grass?
- What do you feed your animals?
- Does any of the feed contain GMOs?
- What are the ingredients in the feed?

I ask that follow-up question because sometimes people are not aware of the hidden GMOs. Therefore, I always ask for an ingredient list so I can check for myself. In my experience, the small farmers are happy to tell you the list of ingredients as well as where they purchase their feed.

If the farmer passes my initial interview, I ask if I can visit their farm. This provides an opportunity to verify the information for myself, to the best of my ability. Besides, it's a fun field trip for the kids. Some farms host a "farm day" where people are welcome to tour their farm and possibly even try free samples of the products they sell. This is a great opportunity to teach your children, from a first-hand perspective, where our food comes from.

You can also support local farmers by joining the Farm-to-Consumer Legal Defense Fund (www.Farmtoconsumer.org). According to their website, the Farm-to-Consumer Legal Defense fund:

- Protects YOUR access to the farmers who feed your family.
- Fights for your farmer's rights in court when the government decides to shut your farmer down.
- Provides legal defense for farmers who are members.

## Grow Your Own

The best way to know what's in the food you eat is to grow your own. Not everyone has acres of land available to grow their own food, but don't let size deter you. You can still grow a small garden even if you live in an apartment. I garden inside using pots during the winter. Garden towers are another option.‡

My son and I have begun gardening in our yard within the past few years, except when I was too sick. Technically, he chases butterflies and catches ladybugs while I pull weeds, but I think that's great. He's involved in the process and that's what is important. Each year he chooses which seeds he wants to plant by reading the seed catalogue (Southern Exposure Seed Exchange; www.southernexposure.com). We

---

‡ For additional information on gardening, including a tool that sends email reminders when it's time to plant crops in your area, visit *Mother Earth News*. The "What to Plant Now" tool can be found at: http://www.motherearthnews. com/organic-gardening/what-to-plant-now-zl0z0903zalt

only buy non-GMO, heirloom seeds. This year he chose to plant sunflower seeds and a melon called "Ice Cream Box." How can you say no to a fruit called "Ice Cream Box?" He knows to only pick organic seeds, preferably heirloom, so that we don't contaminate the Earth with GM plants. He also plants the seeds himself and is in charge of watering the garden. During the growing season, he gives me daily updates on the progress of each plant. We use a ruler to measure their growth and, of course, take pictures along the way.

Because we garden, my son understood the importance of bees by the age of five. He learned that without bees and other pollinators, roughly two-thirds of our crops would be gone.[7] Additionally, in our area, bee colonies have been declining. Once he learned that the bees are in danger, he decided they needed help and it was up to him to save them. Consequently, he began to build bee gardens and track the bees by counting how many came to "drink" from our garden each day. He even asked for a "bee family" for his birthday. We're still contemplating that gift idea!

Growing our own food has changed our relationship with food. I used to throw away enough food to fill an entire grocery bag every couple of weeks. After growing and sourcing our own food, our family now understands how much work it takes to grow healthy food and how much money it costs under our current national food system. Additionally, we have developed a profound appreciation for organic farmers and the effort they put into securing the integrity of our food supply and our natural resources. Consequently, we don't waste food like we used to. Even my son is aware of what foods we can compost so that we can retain those nutrients for our garden. When his cousin comes to visit, my son tells him which foods to put in the compost pile so that we can "feed our garden good nutrients with no bad chemicals."

## Get The Family Involved

No matter what issue I am fighting for, my strategy always begins at home. I like to get the family involved in our food supply, including growing, procuring, and cooking our food. It's important for our children to understand where our food comes from and the work involved in creating and preparing healthy foods. After all, our children will be the stewards of our food supply some day soon. Besides, I realized early in this journey that speaking with our dollars would be a constant power struggle if my family and I were not on the same page.

Not surprisingly, the biggest power struggle was with my husband. Our experience with food has been very different. For instance, at the age of eight, I was taught how to read food labels. My sister and I were only allowed to eat cereal if it did not contain sugar in the first three ingredients. I vividly remember walking down the cereal aisle with my sister, reading the food labels, and trying to find an "acceptable" kids cereal to eat. It was disappointing every time. In addition, I was raised on baked foods, never fried, and no salt added to any of our food. My husband, on the other hand, was raised in an environment where variety meant choosing between Pop-tarts and donuts for breakfast. A hearty helping of vegetables was frozen French fries, which his family would deep fry instead of baking in the oven. Until he was 28, my husband thought wheat was just a flavoring that was added to bread. Needless to say, when I started on the journey of restoring the integrity of our food supply, my husband and I were on opposite ends of the food spectrum.

I've never tried to force my husband to change his diet. I have friends who have tried that approach. From what I've seen, it ends with my friends being frustrated and the men resenting the women for enacting a control grab. As a Libertarian, I'm against forcing anyone to do anything. Consequently, I tried the approach of talking with my husband about the foods he was eating in hopes that he would change his diet on his own accord. That didn't work. Even though I tried to be neutral, I probably came off as judgmental. Besides, people don't want to hear someone telling them they are doing something wrong, especially adults. We had enough lecturing when we were kids. So, I left my husband alone for several months as I wrote this book. Then, one day, everything began to change without me saying a single word.

One day, my husband read the section of my book that talks about the GRAS list. The next day, he went shopping at Costco, which is one of the only errands he likes to do because they have free samples throughout the store. When my husband came home after shopping at Costco that day, he was noticeably irritated. After setting the groceries on the kitchen counter he said to me, "Thanks a lot! You've ruined Costco for me! I looked at some chicken tenders they were passing out and instead of salivating, I got sick to my stomach just looking at them." To which I replied, "Aren't you glad you know and you didn't put that in your body?" His barely audible grunt was not only affirmation for me that my book was effective, it gave us a point of commonality from which we could build. It was our keystone moment that led to my entire family getting involved with our new approach to food, one baby step at a time.

Once our family was onboard, amazing things began to happen. My husband started looking for the Butterfly and only drinking organic milk. I started writing a second book. And my son, at the age of six, created his own cookbook, with my help of course. As I've been teaching him what's in our food supply, he's made the decision not to eat the foods with synthetic chemicals and additives. One day he asked, "Why do other kids eat these foods?" I replied, "Their parents might not know what's in the food they are feeding their children." In that moment, he decided to give kids a choice by making "healthy treats that taste just as good as the treats in the store." Two months later, his dessert line was born: "Rattlesnake Treats: Take the Bite Out of Sweets!" You can find his cookbook at www.HandsOffMyFood.com. Children are amazing! If we get out of their way, there is no limit to the possibilities that lie ahead.

## Make It Affordable

When our family decided to go organic and grain-free, we knew it would be a financial challenge. But, we decided to make it a priority because we see a healthy food supply as an investment in both the immediate and future health of our family.

Consequently, we've adjusted our spending to accommodate the added cost. For example, we no longer eat at restaurants or see movies in the theatre, and I don't go on shopping sprees at the mall. Instead, we cook all of our food at home, wait until movies are available to rent, and buy most of our clothes from garage sales.

In addition, we've found ways to make our food choices more affordable. Here are some ideas that work for us:

- **Buy in bulk:** To decrease the cost, you can buy foods in bulk. For example, I buy bulk containers of shredded coconut and almond flour online. Additionally, some grocery stores allow you to purchase a case of a single food for a discounted price.
- **Buy on sale:** When organic or Non-GMO verified foods are on sale, we stock up. If the foods are perishable, like green beans, I cook them and store them in the freezer in glass containers.

- **Buy from local, uncertified organic farms**: Some farms do practice organic farming but they cannot afford to become USDA organic certified. So, call around to your local farmers and find out if they are using organic farming practices. Some farms allow you to visit the farm and pick your own produce. That option tends to be less expensive and it's a great experience for children.
- **Join a buyer's club**: Discounts are typically offered through buyer's clubs. For example, I belong to the Polyface Farms buyer's club. They routinely offer 'buy one get one free' sales.
- **Avoid the Dirty Dozen:** If you can't afford to eat organic 100% of the time, eat organic when it matters most. Every year the Environmental Working Group releases the "Dirty Dozen," which is a list of the 12 fruits and vegetables containing the most pesticides. When fruits and vegetables are on the Dirty Dozen list, buy the organic version. The list is available at: https://www.ewg.org/foodnews/dirty_dozen_list.php

## Build A Support Group

It's great to have your family on-board, but it also helps to surround yourself with friends who have the same goal. My success as a watchdog over our food supply is highly correlated to having a support system. Fortunately, I am blessed to know like-minded Moms who don't want to feed their kids GMOs, pesticides, chemical additives, and gluten. Having a shared goal allows us to help each other stay on track. For example, we swap recipes that adhere to our goals. And, since all of our kids eat based on the same goals, none of our kids are singled out as the "odd one" for eating "special foods" at picnics and other gatherings. Since we all eat those "special foods," it has become a "normal" way of life for our children and us. There is no teasing, or strange looks. On the contrary, it's just a bunch of kids hanging out and eating foods that all of us Moms feel good about.

Remember the birthday cupcake story I shared earlier in the book? Thanks to my support group of like-minded Moms, I no longer have to worry about chemicals in the cupcakes at those birthday parties. And, when attending parties outside of my support group, my family brings our own dessert. My kids help me bake our cupcakes and decorate them with lots of coconut whip cream and fruit on top. They don't feel like they are missing out because my kids love the taste of our desserts, they love being part of the creative process, and they love how our food makes them feel when they eat it.

## Start A Petition

If you find an ingredient in your favorite processed food that you want removed, start a petition asking the company to remove that ingredient or replace it with an acceptable alternative. For example, artificial dye can be replaced with natural coloring, such as turmeric or paprika.

You can start a petition for free using one of the following websites:
https://www.change.org
http://www.care2.com

## Spread The Word

You can rally support for your cause by engaging your friends and family. Share your passion with them. If it stirs their soul, you now have an ally.

## Stay Informed

To selectively give your consent, you must be informed. Reading this book is a good start! Now it's up to you to build on that information.

Following all the issues with our food supply is time consuming. That's why I sign up for free email alerts from certain groups that follow issues I care about. I don't always agree politically with these groups, but we do share common goals that we can rally behind. Some of these groups include:

- Center for Food Safety (www.centerforfoodsafety.org)
- Environmental Working Group (www.ewg.org)
- Institute for Responsible Technology (www.responsibletechnology.org)
- GM Watch (www.gmwatch.org)
- Natural News (www.naturalnews.com)
- National Resources Defense Council (www.nrdc.org)
- The Food Revolution Network (www.foodrevolution.org)
- U.S. Right to Know (www.usrtk.org)
- Farm-to-Consumer Legal Defense Fund (www.farmtoconsumer.org)

Email alerts typically tell you what action is required, such as signing a petition or emailing your Congressman to vote against a bill. If we don't let our voices be heard, the status quo will remain. It takes less than one minute to respond to an email alert.

## Vote Them Out And In

'Feed the good and starve the bad' also applies to politicians. Use your consent to vote out the politicians who vote for bills that hurt our food supply and vote in candidates who vow to restore its integrity. To find out how your elected officials vote on bills, visit www.GovTrack.us

## Think Local Government

I try not to deal with the federal government whenever possible. Aside from responding to email alerts I receive and helping to keep my friends and family informed, I choose to work with my local community to solve our local problems. Local governments can make huge strides in restoring the integrity of our food. For instance, in 2016, voters in Sonoma County, California, banned GM crops in their county. Measure M (Sonoma County Transgenic Contamination Ordinance) passed with 55.9% of the vote.[8]

Another example of how effective you can be at the local level is rBGH. In the 1990s, over 100 school districts in the United States banned rBGH-milk from their schools.[9] Why? The Parent and Teacher Associations protested. Once mothers found out that the school was feeding their children milk that came from cows treated with a genetically engineered hormone, they banded together and put an end to it. What type of milk does your local school provide children? Does it contain growth hormone? If you don't know, that's a good place to start.

## Take Home Message

We can restore the integrity of our food supply by reclaiming our role as watchdogs. It boils down to using our consent to 'feed the good and starve the bad:'

- Vote with your dollars every time you eat.
- Vote at the ballot box.
- Support third party, independent watchdog groups like the Non-GMO Project and the Environmental Working Group.

Restoring the integrity of our food supply begins at home, one step at a time. Involve the whole family, when possible. Make it fun by cooking with your kids in the kitchen, planting a garden together, or playing the game of looking for the Butterfly during your next trip to the grocery store. Changing our food supply does not have to be a chore. If we take it one day at a time, and work on one goal at a time, together we will build a new mountain.

One thing is for sure: We have modernity on our side. If we tried to restore our food supply thirty or more years ago, it would have been nearly impossible. The Internet has changed all of that. It is the greatest weapon the world has ever seen when it comes to disseminating information and bringing together disparate networks of individuals toward a common goal. Today, we have a way to connect and work together. We have the means necessary to become watchdogs together.

## Moving Forward

Now that you know how to 'feed the good and starve the bad,' let's figure out what *you* are passionate about.

## CHAPTER 12

# WHERE TO BEGIN YOUR FIGHT

Each of us has God-given gifts and passions. It's up to you to figure out what you are passionate about and how you want to fight for it. I've included some ideas in this chapter, but each journey is unique. If you follow your heart and listen to your gut, you won't be led astray.

## Find Your Passion

Decide what is important to you. What are you passionate about? Is there one issue that touches your soul and makes you want to stand up and fight? Your passion may be fighting for better treatment of livestock, or removal of artificial sweeteners from our food supply, or ridding the world of GMOs, or playing one of Bach's symphonies to our crops. Yep, you read that correctly. Plants may be able to "hear." In 2008, a study published in *Molecular Breeding* concluded that rice grew faster when listening to classical music.[1] That may sound like junk science, but it resonates with someone. And, that's the point.

We all have different passions, which is fantastic because that means if we work together, we can restore our food supply. Discover what resonates with you. It's no secret that my passion is GMOs. I'd love for you to join me in that fight, but each of us needs to find our own passion. Once you discover what moves you, you're ready for the next step.

## Be A Detective

Once you have identified your passion, explore it. Become your own detective. Just like Sarah's battle against Gatorade®, or my fight against

GMOs, your fight will probably begin with your own curiosity. Chase it! Let your curiosity lead you on a scavenger hunt where each clue brings you closer to a true understanding of your passion.

Being your own detective can be overwhelming. Often, the hardest part is finding a starting point. So, I try not to overthink it. I simply start with whatever is in front of me. It may be a web article, blog post, scientific journal article, government document, newspaper article, radio or television advertisement, or a conversation with a friend. Maybe your starting point is a phone call to the company who makes your favorite ice cream asking if they use ingredients from cows treated with growth hormones. Whatever your starting point may be, it contains clues that will lead you to your next source. Find those clues and see where they take you. Try to trace the clues all the way back to the original documents or original source, whenever possible.

If you don't have a starting point, another option is to type your passion into a web search and just start reading. Fortunately for us, access to the Internet has made independent exploration simple. You can do most of your research from the convenience of your own home.

No matter where you start, there will be pitfalls to watch out for. So, when I put on my detective hat, I follow these basic guidelines:

1. **Trust your intuition**. We were all given the gift of intuition. Use it. Listen to your gut. When that little red flag rises in your mind, trust it. Follow up on it because you were given that gift of discernment for a reason. You never know where it will lead you. Look what happened when I read my milk label. I followed my instinct and it led to me publishing a book and joining the fight against GMOs! Sarah read her Gatorade® bottle, saw an ingredient that didn't sit right with her, and led an Internet campaign that changed the formulation of Gatorade®! Trust your intuition. It can lead you to do great and impactful things.

2. **Question everything and everyone**. I don't take anyone's word as truth because everyone has an agenda. That doesn't mean I'm cynical. I just know that we all have a natural bias because we're human. I'm not placing judgment on that bias. I am simply acknowledging it exists. My book is biased. That's why I cite my sources. It gives you the opportunity to read the source for yourself and make your own conclusions. Since everyone has a

bias, whenever possible, I find the original documents. I read them and interpret them for myself. I also question the motive of the writer. Whether I'm reading a blog, news article, press release, book, or scientific journal, I always look for the conflicts of interest. An easy way to determine potential bias when reading scientific articles is to look at the author's affiliations. They are often listed directly on the article. Read that disclaimer and decide if you think there is a conflict of interest. Even if there is no conflict of interest indicated in the disclaimer, I still read all scientific articles with a questioning eye. Sometimes the connections between government and industry are omitted from the scientific journal articles. Additionally, we know that many scientists conducting research in the nutrition field are either directly or indirectly chained to industry and/or the government. Personally, I question the findings of any publication that is sponsored by either industry or the government because there is an inherent conflict of interest. Questioning the motive doesn't mean that I don't believe the publication. It means that I find the original source and fact check the publication. If the original source is not available, I try to find a third party, independent publication that can verify or back-up the publication. Regardless, no matter what the source may be, I always approach all publications with an inquisitive eye.

3. **Know all sides of the argument.** That means reading articles and documents that might make you uncomfortable. All resources are biased, so it's our responsibility to collect information from multiple sources and discern the truth for ourselves. Besides, if you get all your information from one source, how will you truly know what you think about the issue? Reading opposing sides helps challenge your beliefs. You will either walk away feeling more convicted in your beliefs or you will have a new perspective to contemplate. Besides, if you only read one side of the argument, how will you know what your opposition thinks? I always try to anticipate what my opponent will say. I do that by reading a variety of sources. It's important to learn what the opposition thinks so you can be ready to defend your issue. So, be prepared and don't let anyone catch you off-guard.

When we are caught off-guard, emotions can take over and that's a quick way to lose your argument.

Once you have educated yourself on your specific passion, discover your core principles.

## Know Your Core Principles

Before you jump in to the fight, I strongly recommend knowing your core principles. If you don't know your core principles, how can you selectively give your consent and, thereby, effectively assert your power? Knowing your core principles will allow you to stay the course during your fight.

> "It matters not where you live, or what rank of life you hold, the evil or the blessing will reach you all. The far and the near, the home counties and the back, the rich and the poor, will suffer or rejoice alike. The heart that feels not now is dead; the blood of his children will curse his cowardice, who shrinks back at a time when a little might have saved the whole, and made them happy. I love the man that can smile in trouble, that can gather strength from distress, and grow brave by reflection. 'Tis the business of little minds to shrink; but he whose heart is firm, and whose conscience approves his conduct, will pursue his principles unto death."
>
> –Thomas Paine, December 23, 1776 ("The Crisis")

On that note, it's easy to say you are against something. It can be difficult to explain *why* you are against something. And, unless you know why you are against something, you can't be grounded in your principles. You'll be susceptible to outside influences and more easily swayed by someone else's agenda. Having core principles roots you in your foundational belief system. According to the 1828 Webster's Dictionary, principle is defined as:

> "the cause, source or origin of any thing; that from which a thing proceeds;...a general truth;...tenet; that which is believed, whether truth or not, but which serves as a rule of action or the basis of a system..."

Principle is what you believe at your core, in your soul. It is what your belief system is based on. Have you ever asked yourself what you stand for? Have you ever thought about *why* you stand for those principles? It's critical to know what you stand for because your actions in life are based on your principles. Thus, if you don't know your core beliefs, it is easy to be misguided or to falter from *your* truth. Trust me, it's easy to get knocked off course when you are not firmly grounded. I found that out the hard way.

When I first learned about GMOs, I did something I am not proud of. My girlfriend sent an email to a group of our friends requesting that we sign a petition in favor of government mandated labeling of all GMO-containing products. I diligently signed the petition and did my part by forwarding it along to my contacts. I felt great! I engaged in the issue and I did something about it. I participated. I was helping to create change. I felt patriotic and empowered. Roughly two hours later, I was knocked off my pedestal.

One of the many people I sent the petition to was my husband's best friend. He promptly called me out on my hypocrisy: I'm a limited government constitutionalist yet I was calling for more government regulation to solve the GMO labeling issue. His email is what prompted me to look into my soul and figure out where I stood on the labeling issue and, consequently, on all issues.

After much deliberation, I firmly knew my core principles:

- Faith in God.
- Love for my neighbors.
- Maximal personal freedom; maximal personal responsibility.

Consequently, I realized that I do not believe in government mandated labeling. I think it's the wrong approach to the problem of GMOs. But, when my girlfriend sent the petition, I acted out of fear. I was not rooted in my core principles. I did not know what I truly stood for. I did not have a strategy to fight against GMOs. I just knew they were bad and I needed to help get rid of them. So, I did what most people do. I stayed on the course that I was taught. I chose the path of relying on government to fix our problems.

Relying on the government was a habit, as well as an easy solution. By demanding that the government be in charge of labeling my foods, I handed the responsibility over to them. I washed my hands of my individual responsibility. It wasn't my problem anymore; it was the government's problem. What I didn't realize at the time was that by signing the petition, I had given my *consent* to the government. And, by giving my consent, I had implicitly given the government the *authority* to fix the problem. I had become part of the problem. I was helping to make the government control of our food supply even bigger, and that is against my core principles. It took a friend to wake me up. Now I'm grateful for the opportunity of hitting rock bottom because it helped me get to know myself. It was my strategic turning point in my journey.

## Ground Yourself

Once you know your core principles, ground yourself so that you will not falter from them. There are many ways you can fix yourself firmly to your principles. Maybe your spouse or friend holds you accountable. Maybe you can do it all on your own. Personally, I choose God. He keeps me accountable. Every time I sit down to write, I pray first. I pray for humility and forgiveness. I pray for my veil to be fully lifted and for God to guide me through each day, showing me how to walk this path with honor, purpose and humility.

## Develop Your Strategy

Once you are grounded in your core principles, you are ready to develop your own strategy. What action are *you* going to take?

- Will you start an online petition, like Sarah?
- Will you write a book, like me?
- Will you lobby Congress?
- Will you get government more involved by asking them to label foods or ban certain food ingredients?
- Will you start purchasing processed foods that carry the Butterfly?
- Will you rally a group of friends together to get milk from rBGH-treated cows removed from your local schools and hospitals?
- Will you start a business selling foods you believe in?

There are many opportunities to get involved. And, every individual's strategy will be different. Pick the one that resonates with you and fight for your passion.

## Take Home Message

Take time to figure out what you are passionate about and then fight for it! If you trust your gut and ground yourself in your core principles, you have a greater chance of staying true to yourself and your cause.

## My Pledge To You

My hope is that one day, each of us will go to the grocery store or a fast food chain and know what we are saying with our dollars. I hope that one day, we will all select our foods based on knowing what's in it, who made it, and whom it supports. Making informed choices is the only way we are going to restore the integrity of our food supply. Industry is not going to fix our food supply and neither is our government. It's up to us, "We the People."

Tackling the issue of our food supply is a true case of David and Goliath. We're up against the food industry, the U.S. government, corporate lobbyists, supposed "experts," and crony capitalism. In addition, because our food supply is so complicated, we are not going to know everything about it. And, that's okay. We don't have to know everything. If we work together, we can each take one bite out of the problem. If we each find our own passion and fight for it, together we can change our food supply. Together we can bring back the integrity of our food, which will ultimately lead to healthier individuals, healthier families, a healthier environment, and restoration of freedoms we have lost.

I've stuck my head in the sand for most of my life. I've relied on other people to fight for our food. It's time to stand on my own two feet. It's time to engage in the fight for the integrity of our food so that our children and grandchildren can have a fighting chance at health, longevity, and freedom. I vow, here and now, to continue to educate myself so I can make informed choices. Nobody said it would be easy. Freedom isn't free. But, if we stand together, we will never be alone.

**I stand with those who believe in individual freedom.**

- I stand with those who agree that Americans should not be un-consenting guinea pigs for chemical companies.
- I stand with those who agree that the government should not decide what's on our dinner plate by picking winners and losers based on special interest groups and backdoor deals.

- I stand with those who agree that companies should not be allowed to dump untested synthetic chemicals into our food while the FDA says it's not their problem.
- I stand with those who agree that "We the People" have the right to know what is in the food we eat, even though industry and the FDA are working hard to keep us in the dark.

### Will you stand with me?

All we have to do is shovel *one* scoop of dirt at a time and eventually we will build a new mountain. We will defeat Goliath. But, it takes that first step. *You* have to pick up the shovel. What do you say? Are you ready to help me build a new mountain?

When you're ready to grab your shovel, I'll be waiting.

### www.HandsOffMyFood.com

# Acronyms

ACS – American Cancer Society (www.cancer.org)

ADA – American Dietetic Association, now called the Academy of Nutrition and Dietetics (www.eatright.org)

ADI – Acceptable Daily Intake

AHA – American Heart Association (www.heart.org)

AMA – American Medical Association (www.ama-assn.org)

bGH – Bovine Growth Hormone

BHA – butylated hydroxyanisole

BHT – butylated hydroxytoluene

*Bt* – Bacillus thuringiensis

BVO – brominated vegetable oil

CDC – Center for Disease Control (www.cdc.gov)

CMAB – California Milk Advisory Board (www.realcaliforniamilk.com)

CRA – Corn Refiners Association (www.corn.org)

CVM – Center for Veterinary Medicine (www.fda.gov/AnimalVeterinary/)

DDT – dichlorodiphenyltrichloroethane

DES – diethylstilbestrol

DNA – deoxyribonucleic acid

EGCG – Epigallocatechin-3-gallate

EMS –     eosinophilia myalgia syndrome

EPA –     Environmental Protection Agency (www.epa.gov)

EWG –     Environmental Working Group (www.ewg.org)

FDA –     U.S. Food and Drug Administration (www.fda.gov)

FDC –     Food, Drug, and Cosmetics

FEMA –    Flavor and Extract Manufacturers Association (www.femaflavor.org)

FTC –     Federal Trade Commission (www.ftc.gov)

GABA –    Gamma-aminobutyric acid

GAO –     Government Accountability Office (www.gao.gov)

GE –      genetically engineered

GM –      genetically modified

GMA –     Grocery Manufacturers Association (www.gmaonline.org)

GMO –     genetically modified organism

GRAS –    generally recognized as safe

HFCS –    high fructose corn syrup

HGH –     human growth hormone

HMF –     hydroxymethylfurfural

IDFA –    International Diary Foods Association (www.idfa.org)

IGF-1 –   Insulin-like Growth Factor-1

JAMA –    Journal of the American Medical Association (www.jamanetwork.com/journals/jama)

NASDA –   National Association of State Departments of Agriculture (www.nasda.org)

NFPA –    National Food Processors Association (www.nfpa-food.org)

NIH –     National Institute for Health (www.nih.gov)

NRDC –    Natural Resources Defense Council (www.nrdc.org)

rBGH –    Recombinant Bovine Growth Hormone

SCOGS –   Select Committee on GRAS Substances

USDA –    United States Department of Agriculture (www.usda.gov)

UV –      Ultraviolet

# TRADEMARK ACKNOWLEDGMENT

All product names, logos, brands, and other trademarks identified or referred to within this book are the property of their respective trademark holders. All company, product, logo, and service names used in the book are for identification purposes only. Use of these names and brands does not imply endorsement.

- Mountain Dew® is a registered trademark of PepsiCo, Inc.
- Chipotle® is a registered trademark of Chipotle Mexican Grill, Inc.
- Tagamet® is a registered trademark of Medtech Products, Inc.
- Oreos® is a registered trademark of Intercontinental Great Brands, LLC.
- Cheetos® is a registered trademark of Frito-Lay North America, Inc.
- Cheez Whiz® is a registered trademark of Kraft Foods Global Brands, LLC.
- Tang® is a registered trademark of Kraft Foods Global Brands, LLC.
- Kraft Macaroni & Cheese® is a registered trademark of Kraft Foods Global Brands, LLC.
- Twinkie® is a registered trademark of Hostess Brands, LLC.
- Sara Lee® is a registered trademark of Sara Lee TM Holdings, LLC.
- Contadina® is a registered trademark of Del Monte Foods, Inc.
- Pop Secret® is a registered trademark of Diamond Foods, Inc.
- Pillsbury® is a registered trademark of The Pillsbury Company, LLC.
- Kix®, Lucky Charms®, Fiber One®, and Cheerios® and are all registered trademarks of General Mills IP Holdings II, LLC.
- Reese's Puffs® is a registered trademark of Hershey Chocolate & Confectionery Corporation.
- Hamburger Helper® is a registered trademark of General Mills, Inc.

- Roundup® and Roundup Ready® are registered trademarks of Monsanto Company.
- NutraSweet® is a registered trademark of NutraSweet Property Holdings, Inc.
- Doritos® is a registered trademark of Frito-Lay North America, Inc.
- Frito-Lay® is a registered trademark of Frito-Lay North America, Inc.
- Gatorade® is a registered trademark of PepsiCo, Inc.
- McDonald's® is a registered trademark of McDonald's Corporation
- Chick-fil-A® is a registered trademark of CFA Properties, Inc.
- Panera® is a registered trademark of Pumpernickel Associates, LLC.
- Dang® is a registered trademark of Dang Foods, LLC.
- Ben & Jerry's® is a registered trademark of Ben & Jerry's Homemade, Inc.
- Hershey's® Kisses® and Milk Chocolate Bar® are a registered trademarks of Hershey Chocolate & Confectionery Corporation
- Campbell's® is a registered trademark of Campbell Soup Company
- Kellogg's® is a registered trademark of Kellogg North America Company
- Mars® is a registered trademark of Mars, Incorporated
- General Mill's® is a registered trademark of General Mills, Inc.
- ConAgra® is a registered trademark of ConAgra, Inc.
- Quaker Oats® is a registered trademark of The Quaker Oats Company
- General Foods® is a registered trademark of General Foods Corporation
- Wonder® Bread is a registered trademark of Flowers Foods, Inc.
- Kool-Aid® is a registered trademark of Kraft Foods Group Brands, LLC.
- Velveeta® is a registered trademark of Kraft Foods Group Brands, LLC.
- Spam® is a registered trademark of Hormel Foods, LLC.
- Crisco® is a registered trademark of The J.M. Smucker Company

# REFERENCES

## Introduction:

1.  United States Food and Drug Administration. CPG Sec. 550.625 Oranges-Artificial Coloring. *fda.gov*. 1980. Available at: http://www.fda. gov/ICECI/ComplianceManuals/CompliancePolicyGuidanceManual/ ucm074540.htm. Accessed August 13, 2016.
2.  Conley M. Flame Retardant in Your Mountan Dew? Yep. *www. abcnews.go.com*. 2011. Available at: http://abcnews.go.com/blogs/ health/2011/12/15/flame-retardant-in-your-mountain-dew-yep/.
3.  Bhasin K. Here's what you need to know about the ground-up insects that Starbucks puts in your Frappuccino. *www.businessinsider. com*. 2012. Available at: http://www.businessinsider.com/ how-cochineal-insects-color-your-food-and-drinks-2012-3/#the-cochineal-insect-is-native-to-mexico-and-south-america-and-contrary-to-the-popular-nomenclature-theyre-not-technically-beetles-theyre-tiny-and-live-on-cactus-plants-usually-the-prickly-pear-cactus-1.
4.  Rivas A. McDonald's Use Of Ammonium Hydroxide To "Wash" Meat Angers Chef Jamie Oliver, But They're Not The Only Culprit. *www. medicaldaily.com*. 2013. Available at: http://www.medicaldaily.com/ mcdonalds-use-ammonium-hydroxide-wash-meat-angers-chef-jamie-oliver-theyre-not-only-249387.
5.  The Oldspeak Journal. 70% Of Ground Beef Contains Ammonia-Soaked "Pink Slime"; USDA Bought 7 Million Pounds For School Lunches. *www.theoldspeakjournal.wordpress. com*. 2012. Available at: https://theoldspeakjournal.wordpress. com/2012/03/13/70-of-ground-beef-contains-ammonia-soaked-pink-slime-usda-bought-7-million-pounds-for-school-lunches/.
6.  The Pew Charitable Trusts. *Fixing the Oversight of Chemicals Added to Our Food: Findings and Recommendations of Pew's Assessments of the U.S. Food Additives Program*. 2013. Available at: http://www.pewtrusts.org/

en/research-and-analysis/reports/2013/11/07/fixing-the-oversight-of-chemicals-added-to-our-food.

7.  Fantozzi J. Common Foods and Drinks Hiding the Antifreeze Compound. *www.thedailymeal.com*. 2014. Available at: http://www.thedailymeal.com/news/common-foods-and-drinks-hiding-antifreeze-compound/103014.

8.  Quilty D. What Is BHT and why you should avoid it. *The Good Human*. 2009.

9.  Anon. Butylated Hydroxytoluene (BHT). *GreenMedInfo*.

10. Kellogg's®. Kellogg's® Froot Loops® cereal. *www.kelloggs.com*. 2016. Available at: https://www.kelloggs.com/en_US/products/kellogg-s-froot-loops-cereal-product.html. Accessed November 11, 2016.

11. Government Accountability Office. *FOOD SAFETY: FDA Should Strengthen Its Oversight of Food Ingredients Determined to Be Generally Recognized as Safe (GRAS)*. 2010:74.

12. GAO. *Recombinant Bovine Growth Hormone: FDA Approval Should Be Withheld Until the Mastitis Issue is Resolved*. 1992:68.

13. Epstein, Samuel, M.D., Cummins, Ronnie, Kinsman, John, Pusztai, Arpad, Smith J. *Petition Seeking the Withdrawal of the New Animal Drug Application Approval for Posilac-Recombinant Bovine Growth Hormone (rBGH)*. 2007.

# Chapter 1:

1.  Wieczner J. Chipotle's "Free Burrito" Coupons Are Making People Less Scared to Eat There. *Fortune*. 2016. Available at: http://fortune.com/2016/03/04/chipotle-coupons-ecoli/.

2.  Dr. Tom O'Bryan. The Gluten Summit. *theglutensummit.com*. 2015. Available at: www.theglutensummit.com. Accessed November 9, 2016.

3.  Dr. Peter Osborne. 43 Facts About Gluten You Might Not Know... *www.glutenfreesociety.org*. 2014. Available at: https://www.glutenfreesociety.org/43-facts-about-gluten-you-might-not-know/. Accessed November 9, 2016.

4.  Leonard M, Vasagar B. US perspective on gluten-related diseases. *Clinical and Experimental Gastroenterology*. 2014;7:25–37. Available at: http://thedr.com/wp-content/uploads/2014/11/US-perspective-on-gluten-related-diseases-Leonard-2014.pdf.

5.  va Berge-Henegouwen G, Mulder C. Pioneer in the gluten free diet: Willem-Karel Dicks 1905-1962, over 50 years of gluten free diet. *Gut*. 1993;34(11):1473–5. Available at: http://www.ncbi.nlm.nih.gov/pubmed/8244125/.

6.  Consumer Reports. How Much Arsenic Is in Your Rice? *www.consumerreports.org*. 2014. Available at: http://www.consumerreports.

org/cro/magazine/2015/01/how-much-arsenic-is-in-your-rice/index. htm. Accessed November 8, 2016.

7. Center for Disease Control. Achievements in Public Health, 1900-1999: Safer and Healthier Foods. *www.cdc.gov*. Available at: https://www.cdc.gov/mmwr/preview/mmwrhtml/mm4840a1.htm. Accessed November 9, 2016.

8. Badii C, Solan M, Reed-Guy L. Beriberi. *www.healthline.com*. 2015. Available at: http://www.healthline.com/health/beriberi#Overview1. Accessed November 9, 2016.

9. Centers for Disease Control and Prevention. Chronic Diseases: The Leading Causes of Death and Disability in the United Stats. *www.cdc.gov*. 2015. Available at: http://www.cdc.gov/chronicdisease/overview/. Accessed September 13, 2016.

10. Olshansky J, Passaro D, Hershow R, et al. A Potential Decline in Life Expectancy in the United States in teh 21st Century. *The New Englad Journal of Medicine*. 2005;352:1138–1145.

11. Centers for Disease Control and Prevention. Heart Disease Facts. *www.cdc.gov*. 2015. Available at: http://www.cdc.gov/heartdisease/facts.htm. Accessed September 23, 2016.

12. National Conference of State Legislatures. *Chronic Disease Prevention and Management*. Denver; 2013. Available at: http://www.ncsl.org/documents/health/chronicdtk13.pdf.

13. Xu J, Murphy S, Kochanek K, Arias E. NCHS Data Brief No. 267: Mortality in the United States, 2016. *www.cdc.gov*. 2016. Available at: http://www.cdc.gov/nchs/data/databriefs/db267.pdf.

14. Centers for Disease Control and Prevention. Cancer. *www.cdc.gov*. 2016. Available at: http://www.cdc.gov/chronicdisease/resources/publications/aag/dcpc.htm. Accessed November 11, 2016.

15. Zimm A. Chronic illnesses on rise, study says Children's cases in US quadruple. *The Boston Globe*. 2007. Available at: http://archive.boston.com/news/nation/articles/2007/06/27/chronic_illnesses_on_rise_study_says/.

16. Perrin JM, Bloom SR, Gortmaker SL. The increase of childhood chronic conditions in the United States. *JAMA : the journal of the American Medical Association*. 2007;297(24):2755–9. Available at: http://apps.webofknowledge.com.ezproxy.fgcu.edu/full_record.do?product=UA&search_mode=Refine&qid=18&SID=2Dipkije2e@L8hHLALi&page=3&doc=21. Accessed October 25, 2012.

17. Johnson R, Segal M, Sautin Y, et al. Potential role of sugar (fructose) in the epidemic of hypertension, obesity and the metabolic syndrome, diabetes, kidney disease, and cardiovascular disease. *The American Journal of Clinical Nutrition*. 2007;86(4):899–906.

18. Adlercreutz H. Western diet and Western diseases: some hormonal and biochemical mechanisms and associations. *Scand J Clin Lab Invest Suppl.* 1990;201:3–23. Available at: https://www.ncbi.nlm.nih.gov/pubmed/2173856.

19. Manzel A, Muller D, Hafler D, et al. Role of "Western Diet" in Inflammatory Autoimmune Disease. *Curr Allergy Asthma Rep.* 2014;14(1):404. Available at: https://www.ncbi.nlm.nih.gov/pubmed/24338487.

20. Cordain L, Eaton B, Sebastian A, et al. Origins and evolution of the Western diet: health implications for 21st century. *The American Journal of Clinical Nutrition.* 2005;81(2):341–354. Available at: http://ajcn.nutrition.org/content/81/2/341.full.

21. Campbell A. Autoimmunity and the Gut. *Autoimmune Diseases.* 2014;152428. Available at: http://doi.org/10.1155/2014/152428.

22. Partnership to Fight Chronic Disease. The Growing Crisis of Chronic Disease in the United States. *www.fightchronicdiseases.org.* Available at: http://www.fightchronicdisease.org/sites/default/files/docs/GrowingCrisisofChronicDiseaseintheUSfactsheet_81009.pdf. Accessed November 11, 2016.

23. Fitzgerald R. *The Hundred-Year Lie: How Food and Medicine Are Destroying Your Health.* New York, NY: Penguin Group; 2006.

24. Unsworth J. History of Pesticide Use. *www.agrochemicals.iupac.org.* 2010. Available at: http://agrochemicals.iupac.org/index.php?option=com_sobi2&sobi2Task=sobi2Details&catid=3&sobi2Id=31.

25. Rosenboro K. Why Is Glyphosate Sprayed on Crops Right Before Harvest? *Ecowatch.com.* 2016. Available at: http://www.ecowatch.com/why-is-glyphosate-sprayed-on-crops-right-before-harvest-1882187755.html.

26. Main D. Glypohsate Now the Most-Used Agricultural Chemical Ever. *www.newsweek.com.* 2016. Available at: http://www.newsweek.com/glyphosate-now-most-used-agricultural-chemical-ever-422419.

27. Hoffman B. GMO Crops Mean More Herbicide, Not Less. *www.forbes.com.* 2013. Available at: http://www.forbes.com/sites/bethhoffman/2013/07/02/gmo-crops-mean-more-herbicide-not-less/#662e48e9a371.

28. Corn + Soybean Digest. Pesticide, herbicide use in U.S. agriculture, 1960-2008. *www.cornandsoybeandigest.com.* 2014. Available at: http://cornandsoybeandigest.com/crop-chemicals/pesticide-herbicide-use-us-agriculture-1960-2008#slide-4-field_images-91381. Accessed November 11, 2016.

29. Fernandez-Cornejo J, Nehring R, Osteen C, et al. *Pesticide Use in U.S. Agriculture: 21 Selected Crops, 1960-2008.* Washington DC;

2014. Available at: https://www.ers.usda.gov/webdocs/publications/
eib124/46734_eib124.pdf.

30. International Agency for Research on Cancer. *IARC Monographs
Volume 112: evaluation of five organophosphate insecticides and herbicides.*
2015:2. Available at: http://www.iarc.fr/en/media-centre/iarcnews/pdf/
MonographVolume112.pdf.

31. Poti JM, Mendez MA, Wen Ng S, Popkin BM. Is the degree of food
processing and convenience linked with the nutritional quality of foods
purchased by US households? *American Journal of Clinical Nutrition.*
2015;101(6). Available at: http://doi.org/10.3945/ajcn.114.100925.

32. U.S. FDA. Statement of Policy-Foods Derived from New Plant
Varieties. *Federal Register.* 1992;57(no. 104).

## Chapter 2:

1. Pesticide Action Network. Children. *www.panna.org.* Available at:
http://www.panna.org/human-health-harms/children. Accessed
November 8, 2016.

2. Bearer CF. Environmental Health Hazards: How Children Are Different
from Adults. *The Future of Children.* 1995;5(2). Available at: https://
www.princeton.edu/futureofchildren/publications/docs/05_02_02.pdf.

3. Adams KM, Lindell KC, Kohlmeier M, Zeisel S. Status of nutrition
education in medical schools. *American Journal of Clinical Nutrition.*
2006;83(4):941S–944S.

4. Ryan T. *Real Food Revolution.* New York City: Hay House, Inc. 2014.

5. The Pew Charitable Trusts. *Fixing the Oversight of Chemicals Added to
Our Food: Findings and Recommendations of Pew's Assessments of the U.S.
Food Additives Program.* 2013. Available at: http://www.pewtrusts.org/
en/research-and-analysis/reports/2013/11/07/fixing-the-oversight-of-
chemicals-added-to-our-food.

6. Poti JM, Mendez MA, Wen Ng S, Popkin BM. Is the degree of food
processing and convenience linked with the nutritional quality of foods
purchased by US households? *American Journal of Clinical Nutrition.*
2015;101(6). Available at: http://doi.org/10.3945/ajcn.114.100925.

7. Smith JM. *Seeds of Deception: Exposing Industry and Government
Lies About the Safety of the Genetically Engineered Foods You're Eating.*
Fairfield, IA: Yes Books; 2003.

8. U.S. FDA. Statement of Policy-Foods Derived from New Plant
Varieties. *Federal Register.* 1992;57(no. 104).

9. FDA. About FDA History. *U.S. Food and Drug Administration Website.*

10. Seife C. Research Misconduct Identified by the US Food and Drug
Administration: Out of Sight, Out of Mind, Out of the Peer-
Reviewed Literature. *JAMA Internal Medicine.* 2015;175(4):567–577.

Available at: http://archinte.jamanetwork.com/article.
aspx?articleid=2109855&resultClick=3.

11. Huff E. Academic oligarchy: Majority of science publishing is controlled by just six companies. *Natural News*. 2015. Available at: http://www.naturalnews.com/050457_science_publishing_academic_oligarchy_corporate_corruption.html.

## Chapter 3:

1. Pillsbury. Funfetti®. *www.pillsburybaking.com*. 2016. Available at: http://www.pillsburybaking.com/products/funfetti/cakes. Accessed November 12, 2016.

2. Center for Science in the Public Interest. *Food Dyes: A Rainbow of Risks*. Washington DC; 2010:1–59. Available at: https://cspinet.org/sites/default/files/attachment/food-dyes-rainbow-of-risks.pdf.

3. Weiss B, Williams J, Margen S, et al. Behavioral responses to artificial food colors. *Science*. 1980;207(4438):1487–1489. Available at: http://science.sciencemag.org/content/207/4438/1487.article-info.

4. Schab D, Trinh N. Do artificial food colors promote hyperactivity in children with hyperactive syndromes? A meta-analysis of double-blind placebo-controlled trials. *Journal of Developmental & Behavioral Pediatrics*. 2004;25(6):423–34. Available at: https://www.ncbi.nlm.nih.gov/pubmed/15613992.

5. McCann D, Barrett A, Cooper A, Crumpler D, Al. E. Food additives and hyperactive behaviour in 3-year-old and 8/9-year-old children in the community: a randomised, double-blinded, placebo-controlled trial. *The Lancet*. 2007;370(9598):1560–1567. Available at: http://www.thelancet.com/journals/lancet/article/PIIS0140673607613063/abstract.

6. Sasaki YF, Kawaguchi S, Kamaya A, et al. The comet assay with 8 mouse organs: Results with 39 currently used food additives. *Mutation Research-Genetic Toxicology and Environmental Mutagenesis*. 2002;519(1-2):103–119.

7. Lancaster F, Lawrence J. Determination of total non-sulphonated aromatic amines in tartrazine, sunset yellow FCF and allura red by reduction and derivatization followed by high-performance liquid chromatography. *Food Additives and Contaminants*. 1991;8(3):249–63. Available at: https://www.ncbi.nlm.nih.gov/pubmed/1778264.

8. Goldschmidt V. 12 Dangerous And Hidden Food Ingredients In Seemingly Healthy Foods. *www.saveourbones.com*. 2016. Available at: https://saveourbones.com/12-dangerous-ingredients/. Accessed November 12, 2016.

9. Lim T, Poole R, Pageler N. Propylene glycol toxicity in children. *J Pediatr Pharmacol Ther*. 2014;19(4):277–282. Available at: https://www.ncbi.nlm.nih.gov/pubmed/25762872.

10. Oikawa S, Nishino K, Inoue S, Mizutani T, Kawanishi S. Oxidative DNA damage and apoptosis induced by metabolites of butylated hydroxytoluene. *Biochem PHarmacol*. 1998;56(3):361–370. Available at: https://www.ncbi.nlm.nih.gov/pubmed/9744574.

11. Bauer A, Dwyer-Nield L, Hankin J, Murphy R, Malkinson A. The lung tumor promoter, butylated hydroxytoluene (BHT), causes chronic inflammation in promotion-sensitive BALB/cByJ mice but not in promotion-resistant CXB4 mice. *Toxicology*. 2001;169(1):1–15. Available at: https://www.ncbi.nlm.nih.gov/pubmed/11696405.

12. Bauer K, Dwyer-Nield L, Keil K, Koski K, Malkinson A. Butylated hydroxytoluene (BHT) induction of pulmonary inflammation: a role in tumor promotion. *Exp Lung Res*. 2001;27(3):197–216. Available at: https://www.ncbi.nlm.nih.gov/pubmed/11293324.

13. Mikkelsen H, Larsen J, Tarding F. Hypersensitivity reactions to food colours with special reference to the natural colour annatto extract (butter colour). *Archives of Toxicology Supplementation*. 1978;1:141–3. Available at: https://www.ncbi.nlm.nih.gov/pubmed/150265.

14. Be Food Smart. Polysorbate 60. *www.befoodsmart.com*. 2011. Available at: http://www.befoodsmart.com/ingredients/polysorbate-60.php. Accessed November 12, 2016.

15. Conley M. Flame Retardant in Your Mountain Dew? Yep. *www.abcnews.go.com*. 2011. Available at: http://abcnews.go.com/blogs/health/2011/12/15/flame-retardant-in-your-mountain-dew-yep/.

16. Frito-Lay. DORITOS® Nacho Cheese Flavored Tortilla Chips. *www.fritolay.com*. 2016. Available at: http://www.fritolay.com/snacks/product-page/doritos/doritos-nacho-cheese-flavored-tortilla-chips. Accessed November 13, 2016.

17. Young F. Disodium Inosinate Side Effects. *www.ehow.com*. Available at: http://www.ehow.com/facts_6828039_disodium-inosinate-side-effects.html. Accessed November 13, 2016.

18. Kruse J. MSG, your GUT, and your BRAIN, Post-Trauma. *www.jackkruse.com*. 2011. Available at: https://www.jackkruse.com/msg-your-gut-and-your-brain-post-trauma/.

19. Kresser C. Beyond MSG: Could Hidden Sources of Glutamate Be Harming Your Health? *www.chriskresser.com*. 2014. Available at: https://chriskresser.com/beyond-msg-could-hidden-sources-of-glutamate-be-harming-your-health/.

20. Zeratsky K. What is MSG? Is it bad for you? *www.mayoclinic.com*. 2015. Available at: http://www.mayoclinic.org/healthy-lifestyle/nutrition-and-healthy-eating/expert-answers/monosodium-glutamate/faq-20058196. Accessed November 13, 2016.

21. Meldrum B. Glutamate as a neurotransmitter in the brain: review of physiology and pathology. *Journal of Nutrition*. 2000;130(4S

Supplement):1007S–15S. Available at: https://www.ncbi.nlm.nih.gov/pubmed/10736372.

22. Schwarcz R, Foster A, French E, Whetsell W, Kohler C. Excitotoxic models for neurodegenerative disorders. *Life Sciences*. 1984;35(1):19–32. Available at: https://www.ncbi.nlm.nih.gov/pubmed/6234446.

23. Rothman S, Olney J. Glutamate and the pathophysiology of hypoxic--ischemic brain damage. *Annals of Neurology*. 1986;19(2):105–11. Available at: https://www.ncbi.nlm.nih.gov/pubmed/2421636.

24. Raiten D, Talbot J, Fisher K. Executive Summary from the Report: Analysis of Adverse Reactions to Monosodium Glutamate (MSG). *The Journal of Nutrition*. 1995;125(11):2891S–2906S. Available at: http://jn.nutrition.org/content/125/11/2891S.extract.

25. Olney J, Sharpe L. Brain lesions in an infant rhesus monkey treated with monsodium glutamate. *Science*. 1969;166(3903):386–8. Available at: https://www.ncbi.nlm.nih.gov/pubmed/5812037.

26. Feder D. Alternatives for MSG. *www.foodprocessing.com*. 2005. Available at: http://www.foodprocessing.com/articles/2005/517/. Accessed November 13, 2016.

27. Hennessy M. Rosemary extract sees "substantial growth" in shelf extension. *www.foodnavigator-usa.com*. 2013. Available at: http://www.foodnavigator-usa.com/Suppliers2/Rosemary-extract-sees-substantial-growth-in-shelf-extension.

28. Frito-Lay. New Year Brings Required Trans Fat Labeling On Nutrition Fact Panel. *www.fritolay.com*. 2005. Available at: http://www.fritolay.com/company/media/media-article/new-year-brings-required-trans-fat-labeling-on-nutrition-fact-panel.

29. Bloom R. Frito-Lay knocks chips off the trans-fatty block. *www.theglobeandmail.com*. 2004. Available at: http://www.theglobeandmail.com/life/frito-lay-knocks-chips-off-the-trans-fatty-block/article994513/.

30. Frito-Lay North America I. News Release: Lay's Potato Chips Cuts Saturated Fat By More Than Half. *News Release*. 2006. Available at: http://phx.corporate-ir.net/phoenix.zhtml?c=78265&p=irol-newsArticle&ID=851367&highlight. Accessed December 18, 2016.

31. Lincoln A. The Gettysburg Address. *www.abrahamlincolnonline.org*. 1863. Available at: http://www.abrahamlincolnonline.org/lincoln/speeches/gettysburg.htm. Accessed September 13, 2016.

32. The Pew Charitable Trusts. *Fixing the Oversight of Chemicals Added to Our Food: Findings and Recommendations of Pew's Assessments of the U.S. Food Additives Program*. 2013. Available at: http://www.pewtrusts.org/en/research-and-analysis/reports/2013/11/07/fixing-the-oversight-of-chemicals-added-to-our-food.

33. Keefe D. Agency Response Letter GRAS Notice No. GRN 000567. *U.S. Food and Drug Administration Website*. 2015. Available at:

http://www.fda.gov/Food/IngredientsPackagingLabeling/GRAS/
NoticeInventory/ucm449888.htm. Accessed July 8, 2015.

34.  U.S. FDA. Statement of Policy-Foods Derived from New Plant Varieties. *Federal Register*. 1992;57(no. 104). Available at: http://www.fda.gov/ Food/GuidanceRegulation/GuidanceDocumentsRegulatoryInformation/ Biotechnology/ucm096095.htm.

35.  Seaman A. Industry influence found in food additive report. *Reuters Health*. 2013. Available at: http://www.reuters.com/article/us-influence-food-additive-idUSBRE9760MZ20130807.

36.  U.S. Department of Health and Human Services Food and Drug Administration Center for Food Safety and Applied Nutrition. *Guidance for Industry: Considerations Regarding Substances Added to Foods, Including Beverages and Dietary Supplements.* 2014:5. Available at: http://www.fda.gov/downloads/Food/ GuidanceRegulation/GuidanceDocumentsRegulatoryInformation/ IngredientsAdditivesGRASPackaging/UCM381316.pdf.

37.  Haspel T. Farm bill: Why don't taxpayers subsidize the foods that are better for us? *The Washington Post*. 2014. Available at: https:// www.washingtonpost.com/lifestyle/food/farm-bill-why-dont-taxpayers-subsidize-the-foods-that-are-better-for-us/2014/02/14/ d7642a3c-9434-11e3-84e1-27626c5ef5fb_story.html.

38.  United States Department of Agriculture Economic Research Service. Corn Background. *ers.usda.gov*. 2016. Available at: http://www.ers.usda. gov/topics/crops/corn/background.aspx. Accessed July 28, 2016.

39.  Edwards C. Agricultural Subsidies. *downsizinggovernment.org*. 2009. Available at: http://www.downsizinggovernment.org/agriculture/ subsidies. Accessed August 26, 2015.

40.  Siegel KR, McKeever-Bullard K, Imperatore G, et al. Association of Higher Consumption of Foods Derived From Subsidized Commodities With Adverse Cardiometabolic Risk Among US Adults. *JAMA Internal Medicine*. 2016;176(8):1124–1132. Available at: http://archinte. jamanetwork.com/article.aspx?articleid=2530901.

41.  Van Hoesen S, Secretary P. How Crop Subsidies May Make You Fat. *ewg.org*. 2016. Available at: http://www.ewg.org/agmag/2016/07/how-crop-subsidies-make-you-fat.

42.  Schiff A. The Supreme Court Still Thinks Corporations Are People. *www.theatlantic.com*. 2012. Available at: http://www.theatlantic.com/ politics/archive/2012/07/the-supreme-court-still-thinks-corporations-are-people/259995/.

43.  Supreme Court of The United States. Citizens United v. Federal Election Commission. 2009;No. 08-205. Available at: https://www. supremecourt.gov/opinions/09pdf/08-205.pdf.

44. Statista. Sales of the leading tortilla and tostada chip brands of the United States in 2016 (in million U.S. dollars). *www.statista.com*. 2016. Available at: https://www.statista.com/statistics/188233/top-tortilla-tostada-chip-brands/. Accessed November 13, 2016.

45. The Healthology. Doritos: The Most Popular Snack That Is Linked to Cancer and Other Diseases. *www.thehealthology.com*. 2016. Available at: http://thehealthology.com/2016/08/doritos-popular-snack-cancer/. Accessed November 13, 2016.

46. Smith JM. *Seeds of Deception: Exposing Industry and Government Lies About the Safety of the Genetically Engineered Foods You're Eating.* Fairfield, IA: Yes Books; 2003.

47. Nestle M. McDonald's goes non-GM (in the U.K., at least). *www.foodpolitics.com*. 2009. Available at: http://www.foodpolitics.com/2009/09/mcdonalds-goes-non-gm-in-the-u-k-at-least/. Accessed September 11, 2016.

## Chapter 4:

1. Fitzgerald R. *The Hundred-Year Lie: How Food and Medicine Are Destroying Your Health.* New York, NY: Penguin Group; 2006.

2. FDA. About FDA History. *U.S. Food and Drug Administration Website*.

3. United States Department of Health & Human. FDA, USDA, NOAA Statements on Food Safety. *www.fda.gov*. 2011. Available at: http://www.fda.gov/NewsEvents/PublicHealthFocus/ucm248257.htm. Accessed September 13, 2016.

4. Schweikart L. *What Would The Founders Say?* New York: Penguin Group; 2011.

5. Swann J. FDA's Origin. *www.fda.gov*. 2014. Available at: http://www.fda.gov/AboutFDA/WhatWeDo/History/Origin/ucm124403.htm. Accessed November 13, 2016.

6. Hilts PJ. The FDA At Work-Cutting-Edge Science Promoting Public Health. *FDA Consumer Magazine*. 2006. Available at: http://www.fda.gov/aboutfda/whatwedo/history/overviews/ucm109801.htm. Accessed June 28, 2016.

7. Meadows M. A Century of Ensuring Safe Foods and Cosmetics. *FDA Consumer Magazine*. 2006.

8. FDA. Significant Dates in U.S. Food and Drug Law History. *FDA*.

9. Levenstein H. *Fear of Food: A History of Why We Worry about What We Eat.* Chicago: The University of Chicago Press; 2012.

10. Schlosser E. "I Aimed For The Public"s Heart, And...hit It In The Stomach'. *Chicago Tribune*. 2006.

11. www.crf-usa.org. Upton Sinclair's The Jungle: Muckraking the Meat-Packing Industry. *Constitutional Rights Foundation*. 2008. Available at: http://www.crf-usa.org/bill-of-rights-in-action/

bria-24-1-b-upton-sinclairs-the-jungle-muckraking-the-meat-packing-industry.html. Accessed June 27, 2016.

12. Cherny RW. The Jungle and the Progressive Era. *The Gilder Lehrman Institute of American History*. Available at: http://www.gilderlehrman. org/history-by-era/politics-reform/essays/jungle-and-progressive-era. Accessed June 28, 2016.

13. Sinclair U. *The Jungle*. Dover Thri. (Negri P, Pine J, eds.). Mineola: Dover Publications, Inc. 2001.

14. Carpenter DP. Pure Food and Drug Act (1906). *Encyclopedia.com*. 2004. Available at: http://www.encyclopedia.com/topic/Food_and_Drug_Act_of_1906.aspx. Accessed June 28, 2016.

15. Tucker JA. When Government Spreads Disease: The 1906 Meat Inspection Act. *Foundation for Economic Education*. 2014. Available at: https://fee.org/articles/when-government-spreads-disease-the-1906-meat-inspection-act/. Accessed June 29, 2016.

16. United States Department of Agriculture. Food Product Dating. *www.fsis.usda.gov*. 2015. Available at: http://www.fsis.usda.gov/wps/portal/fsis/topics/food-safety-education/get-answers/food-safety-fact-sheets/food-labeling/food-product-dating/food-product-dating. Accessed November 13, 2016.

17. Pasour EC. We Can Do Better than Government Inspection of Meat. *Foundation for Economic Education*. 1998. Available at: https://fee.org/articles/we-can-do-better-than-government-inspection-of-meat/. Accessed June 29, 2016.

18. Reed L. Upton Sinclair's "The Jungle" Proved Regulation Was Required. *Foundation for Economic Education*. 2014. Available at: https://fee.org/articles/29-upton-sinclairs-the-jungle-proved-regulation-was-required/. Accessed June 29, 2016.

19. Teicholz N. *The Big Fat Surprise: Why Butter, Meat & Cheese Belong in a Healthy Diet*. New York, NY: Simon & Schuster Paperbacks; 2014.

20. Analysis O of B and P. USDA FY 2017 Budget Summary. *usda.gov*. 2016. Available at: http://www.obpa.usda.gov/budsum/fy17budsum.pdf. Accessed September 26, 2016.

21. U.S. Food and Drug Administration. Title 21-Part 81: General Specifications and Genearl Restrictions for Provisional Color Additives for use in Foods, Drus, and Cosmetics. *Code of Federal Regulations*. 2016;Title 21(Volume 1).

22. United States Department of Agriculture FS and IS. Inspection & Grading of Meat and Poultry: What Are the Differences? *www.fsis.usda.gov*. 2014. Available at: https://www.fsis.usda.gov/wps/portal/fsis/topics/food-safety-education/get-answers/food-safety-fact-sheets/production-and-inspection/

inspection-and-grading-of-meat-and-poultry-what-are-the-differences_/
inspection-and-grading-differences. Accessed December 17, 2016.

23. Rouse KL. Meat Inspection Act of 1906. *Encyclopedia Britannica*. 2016. Available at: http://www.britannica.com/topic/Meat-Inspection-Act. Accessed June 24, 2016.

24. History A& AUSH of R. The Pure Food and Drug Act. *history.house.gov*.

25. Wade LC. Meatpacking. *Encyclopedia of Chicago*. 2005. Available at: http://www.encyclopedia.chicagohistory.org/pages/804.html. Accessed June 28, 2016.

26. Linnekin BJ. The Food-Safety Fallacy: More Regulation Doesn't Necessarily Make Food Safer. *Northeastern University Law Journal*. 2012;4(1).

27. U.S.Department of Agriculture. Faces of Food Safety: Nonnie Holliman. *www.fsis.usda.gov*. 2013. Available at: http://www.fsis.usda. gov/wps/portal/informational/aboutfsis/faces-of-food-safety/faces-food-safety-nhollliman. Accessed June 29, 2016.

28. News Desk. FDA to Withdraw Approval for Arsenic-Based Drug Used in Poultry. *www.foodsafetynews.com*. 2015. Available at: http://www. foodsafetynews.com/2015/04/fda-to-withdraw-approval-for-arsenic-based-drug-used-in-poultry/#.WCi2-Df7blI.

29. The Daily Meal. These American Meat Products Are Banned Abroad. *www.huffingtonpost.com*. 2014. Available at: http://www.huffingtonpost. com/the-daily-meal/these-american-meat-produ_b_5153275.html.

30. Reed L. Of Meat and Myth. *Foundation for Economic Education*. 2013. Available at: https://fee.org/articles/of-meat-and-myth/.

31. Beck G. *Dreamers and Deceivers: True Stories of the Heroes and Villains who made America*. Mercury Radio Arts, Inc. 2014.

32. United States Department of Agriculture Food Safety and Inspection Service. *Safe and Suitable Ingredients Used in the Production of Meat, Poultry, and Egg Products*. Washington DC; 2016.

33. Michael Farris. Personal Communication.

34. Blum D. The Chemist's War. *Slate*. 2010. Available at: http://www. slate.com/articles/health_and_science/medical_examiner/2010/02/ the_chemists_war.html. Accessed June 28, 2016.

35. Federal Register. The Constitutional Amendment Process. *National Archives*. Available at: https://www.archives.gov/federal-register/ constitution/. Accessed June 26, 2016.

36. Anon. Prohibition. *Rustycans.com*. Available at: http://www.rustycans. com/HISTORY/prohibition.html. Accessed June 29, 2015.

## Chapter 5:

1. History Channel. New Deal. *www.History.com*. Available at: http:// www.history.com/topics/new-deal. Accessed July 10, 2016.

2.  National Sustainable Agriculture Coalition. What is the Farm Bill? *www.sustainableagriculture.ent*. Available at: http://sustainableagriculture.net/our-work/campaigns/fbcampaign/what-is-the-farm-bill/. Accessed August 3, 2015.

3.  MacDonald JM, Korb P, Hoppe RA. *Farm Size and the Organization of U.S. Crop Farming*. 2013.

4.  Merino N. *Agricultural Subsidies: Opposing Viewpoints*. (Merino N, ed.). Nasso, Christine; 2010.

5.  Van Hoesen S, Secretary P. How Crop Subsidies May Make You Fat. *ewg.org*. 2016. Available at: http://www.ewg.org/agmag/2016/07/how-crop-subsidies-make-you-fat.

6.  United States Department of Agriculture ERS. Crops. *www.ers.usda.gov*. 2016. Available at: https://www.ers.usda.gov/topics/crops/. Accessed December 18, 2016.

7.  National Oceanic and Atmospheric Administration. Feeds for Aquaculture. *www.nmfs.noaa.gov*. Available at: http://www.nmfs.noaa.gov/aquaculture/faqs/faq_feeds.html#1what. Accessed December 17, 2016.

8.  United States Department of Agriculture Economic Research Service. Corn Background. *ers.usda.gov*. 2016. Available at: http://www.ers.usda.gov/topics/crops/corn/background.aspx. Accessed July 28, 2016.

9.  United States Department of Agriculture ERS. Corn: Background. *www.ers.usda.gov*. 2016. Available at: https://www.ers.usda.gov/topics/crops/corn/background/. Accessed December 17, 2016.

10. Rippe J. *Fructose, High Fructose Corn Syrup, Sucrose and Health*. (Bendich A, ed.). Orlando: Humana Press; 2014.

11. Select Committee on GRAS Substances. Select Committee on GRAS Substances (SCOGS) Opinion: Corn Sugar (Dextrose), Corn Syrup, Invert Sugar. *www.fda.gov*. 1976. Available at: http://www.fda.gov/Food/IngredientsPackagingLabeling/GRAS/SCOGS/ucm261263.htm. Accessed December 17, 2016.

12. Schoonover H, Muller M. *Food without Thought: How U.S. Farm Policy Contributes to Obesity*. 2006. Available at: http://www.iatp.org/files/421_2_80627.pdf.

13. United States Department of Agriculture. Profiling Food Consumption in America. In: *Agriculture Fact Book*.; 2003. Available at: http://www.usda.gov/documents/usda-factbook-2001-2002.pdf.

14. Duffey K, Popkin B. High-Fructose Corn Syrup: Is this what's for dinner? *American Journal of Clinical Nutrition*. 2008;88(6):1722S–1732S.

15. Poti JM, Mendez MA, Wen Ng S, Popkin BM. Is the degree of food processing and convenience linked with the nutritional quality of foods purchased by US households? *American Journal of Clinical Nutrition*. 2015;101(6). Available at: http://doi.org/10.3945/ajcn.114.100925.

16. Frykholm A. Down on the Farm: The problem with Government Subsidies. *ChristianCentury.org*. 2008. Available at: http://www.christiancentury.org/article/2008-04/down-farm.

17. United States Department of Agriculture Economic Research Service. Sugar & Sweeteners Policy. *usda.gov*. 2015. Available at: http://www.ers.usda.gov/topics/crops/sugar-sweeteners/policy.aspx. Accessed July 20, 2016.

18. Griswold D, Slivinski S, Preble C. Six Reasons to Kill Farm Subsidies and Trade Barriers. *Reason.com*. 2006. Available at: http://reason.com/archives/2006/02/01/six-reasons-to-kill-farm-subsi.

19. Edwards C. Agricultural Subsidies. *downsizinggovernment.org*. 2009. Available at: http://www.downsizinggovernment.org/agriculture/subsidies. Accessed August 26, 2015.

20. Fitzgerald R. *The Hundred-Year Lie: How Food and Medicine Are Destroying Your Health*. New York, NY: Penguin Group; 2006.

21. Pollan M. *Omnivore's Dilemma: A Natural History of Fourl Meals*. New York: The Penguin Press; 2006.

22. United States Department of Agriculture Economic Research Service. Soybeans & Oil Crops. *ers.usda.gov*. 2016. Available at: http://www.ers.usda.gov/topics/crops/soybeans-oil-crops/background.aspx. Accessed July 28, 2016.

23. Gupta S. If we are what we eat, Americans are corn and soy. *CNN.com*. Available at: http://www.cnn.com/2007/HEALTH/diet.fitness/09/22/kd.gupta.column/. Accessed July 17, 2016.

24. United States Department of Agriculture; Economic Research Service. Recent Trends in GE Adoption. *www.ers.usda.gov*. 2016. Available at: https://www.ers.usda.gov/data-products/adoption-of-genetically-engineered-crops-in-the-us/recent-trends-in-ge-adoption.aspx. Accessed December 17, 2016.

25. Fernandez-Cornejo J, Wechsler S, Livingston M, Mitchell L. *Genetically Engineered Crops in the United States*. 2014. Available at: http://www.ers.usda.gov/media/1282246/err162.pdf.

26. Siegel KR, McKeever-Bullard K, Imperatore G, et al. Association of Higher Consumption of Foods Derived From Subsidized Commodities With Adverse Cardiometabolic Risk Among US Adults. *JAMA Internal Medicine*. 2016;176(8):1124–1132. Available at: http://archinte.jamanetwork.com/article.aspx?articleid=2530901.

27. Centers for Disease Control and Prevention. Chronic Disease Overview. *cdc.gov*. 2016. Available at: http://www.cdc.gov/chronicdisease/overview/. Accessed August 1, 2016.

28. Cordain L, Eaton B, Sebastian A, et al. Origins and evolution of the Western diet: health implications for 21st century. *The American Journal*

*of Clinical Nutrition.* 2005;81(2):341–354. Available at: http://ajcn.
nutrition.org/content/81/2/341.full.

29. Manzel A, Muller D, Hafler D, et al. Role of "Western Diet" in
Inflammatory Autoimmune Disease. *Curr Allergy Asthma Rep.*
2014;14(1):404. Available at: https://www.ncbi.nlm.nih.gov/
pubmed/24338487.

30. Severson K. Obesity "a threat" to U.S. security/Surgeon general urges
cultural shift. *SFGate.* 2003. Available at: http://www.sfgate.com/
health/article/Obesity-a-threat-to-U-S-security-Surgeon-2686994.php.

31. Pace G. Obesity Bigger Threat Than Terrorism? *CBSNews.* 2006.
Available at: http://www.cbsnews.com/news/obesity-bigger-threat-than-
terrorism/.

32. Nestle M. The farm bill drove me insane. *Politico.* 2016. Available at:
http://www.politico.com/agenda/story/2016/03/farm-bill-congress-
usda-food-policy-000070.

33. Bittman M. *A Bone to Pick: The good and bad news about food, with
wisdom and advice on diets, food safety, GMOs, farming and more.* New
York: Pam Krauss Books; 2015.

34. Nestle M. Food Politics. *Foodpolitics.com.* 2012. Available at: http://
www.foodpolitics.com/tag/price-of-food/. Accessed August 5, 2015.

35. Ryan T. *Real Food Revolution.* New York City: Hay House, Inc. 2014.

36. Pollan M. You Are What You Grow. *The New York Times Magazine.*
2007. Available at: http://michaelpollan.com/articles-archive/you-are-
what-you-grow/.

37. U.S. Food and Drug Administration. Draft Guidance for Industry:
Inorganic Arsenic in Rice Cereals for Infants: Action Level. *fda.gov.*
2016. Available at: http://www.fda.gov/Food/GuidanceRegulation/
GuidanceDocumentsRegulatoryInformation/ucm486305.htm.
Accessed July 29, 2016.

38. Hughes M, Beck B, Chen Y, Lewis A, Thomas D. Arsenic Exposure
and Toxicology: A Historical Perspective. *Toxicological Sciences.*
2011;123(2):305–332.

39. The Dr. Oz Show. Breaking News: FDA Confirms Concerning Arsenic
Levels in Rice. *doctoroz.com.* 2012. Available at: http://www.doctoroz.
com/article/breaking-news-FDA-arsenic-rice. Accessed July 29, 2016.

40. U.S. Food and Drug Administration. Arsenic in Rice and Rice
Products. *fda.gov.* 2016. Available at: http://www.fda.gov/Food/
FoodborneIllnessContaminants/Metals/ucm319870.htm. Accessed July
29, 2016.

41. Block G. Foods contributing to energy intake in the US: data from
NHANES III and NHANES 1999-2000. *Journal of Food Composition
and Analysis.* 2004;17(3-4).

42. United States Department of Agriculture Economic Research Service. Dairy Data Overview. *ers.usda.gov*. 2016. Available at: http://www.ers.usda.gov/data-products/dairy-data.aspx. Accessed July 29, 2016.

43. Mulvany L. The U.S. Is Producing a Record Amount of Milk and Dumping the Leftovers. *Bloomberg*. 2015. Available at: http://www.bloomberg.com/news/articles/2015-07-01/milk-spilled-into-manure-pits-as-supplies-overwhelm-u-s-dairies.

44. The Week Staff. Farm subsidies: A welfare program for agribusiness. *theweek.com*. 2013. Available at: http://theweek.com/articles/461227/farm-subsidies-welfare-program-agribusiness.

45. Riedl B. Seven Reasons to Veto the Farm Bill. *heritage.org*. 2008. Available at: http://www.heritage.org/research/reports/2008/05/seven-reasons-to-veto-the-farm-bill.

46. Stiglitz JE. The Insanity of Our Food Policy. *The New York Times: The Opinion Pages*. 2013. Available at: http://www.aae.wisc.edu/aae375/sustainable_ag/Readings NET/The Insanity of Our Food Policy 2-NYTimes.com.pdf.

47. Mittal A. Free Trade Doesn't Help Agriculture. *fpif.org*. 2007. Available at: http://fpif.org/free_trade_doesnt_help_agriculture/.

48. Coburn TA. *Subsidies of the Rich and Famous: A Report by Tom A. Coburn, M.D.; U.S. Senator, Oklahoma*. 2011. Available at: http://big.assets.huffingtonpost.com/SubsidiesoftheRichandFamous.pdf.

49. The Guardian. Bruce Springsteen and Jon Bon Jovi face big tax bills after New Jersey law change. *theguardian.com*. 2015. Available at: https://www.theguardian.com/music/2015/mar/25/bruce-springsteen-jon-bon-jovi-tax-bills-after-new-jersey-law-change.

50. Government Accountability Office. *Federal Farm Programs: USDA Needs to Strengthen Controls to Prevent Improper Payments to Estates and Deceased Individuals*. 2007.

51. Morgan D, Gaul G, Cohen S. Farm Program Pays $1.3 Billion to People Who Don't Farm. *The Washington Post*. 2006. Available at: http://www.washingtonpost.com/wp-dyn/content/article/2006/07/01/AR2006070100962.html.

52. Riedl BM. How Farm Subsidies Harm Taxpayers, Consumers, and Farmers, Too. *heritage.org*. 2007. Available at: http://www.heritage.org/research/reports/2007/06/how-farm-subsidies-harm-taxpayers-consumers-and-farmers-too#_ftn26. Accessed August 28, 2015.

53. Editorial Board. This farm bill deserves a veto. *The Washington Post*. 2014. Available at: https://www.washingtonpost.com/opinions/this-farm-bill-deserves-a-veto/2014/01/29/4763fd80-8904-11e3-833c-33098f9e5267_story.html.

54. Congress. *Agricultural Adjustment Ace of 1933: Ch. 25, 48 Stat. 31*. Washington DC: United States Congress; 1933. Available at: http://nationalaglawcenter.org/wp-content/uploads/assets/farmbills/1933.pdf.

55. Oxfam America. Fairness in the Fields: A Vision for the 2007 Farm Bill. *OxfamAmerica.org*. 2007. Available at: https://www.oxfamamerica.org/static/media/files/fairness-in-the-fields.pdf. Accessed July 29, 2016.

56. Schweikart L, Allen M. *A Patriot's History of the United States*. New York: Penguin Group; 2004.

57. Ganzel B. AAA, Agricultural Adjustment Act. *www.livinghistoryfarm.org*. 2003. Available at: http://www.livinghistoryfarm.org/farminginthe30s/water_11.html. Accessed June 19, 2016.

58. Michael Farris. Personal Communication.

59. Baumgartner R. Agricultural Adjustment Act 1933 & United States Housing Authority 1937. *Prezi.com*. 2014. Available at: https://prezi.com/krwm9ulhwm4v/copy-of-agricultural-adjustment-act-1933/. Accessed August 26, 2015.

60. Roberts J. United States v. Butler et al., Receivers of Hoosac Mills Corp. No. 401. 1936;297 U.S. 1. Available at: https://scholar.google.com/scholar_case?case=1427345954995665703&q=United+States+v.+Butler,+297+U.S.+1+(1936)&hl=en&as_sdt=6,47&as_vis=1.

61. Economic Research Service. *History of Agricultural Price-Support and Adjustment Programs, 1933-84*. Washington DC; 1984:52.

62. Nestle M. The farm bill promotes fruits and vegetables? Really? *Foodpolitics.com*. 2014. Available at: http://www.foodpolitics.com/tag/farm-bill/. Accessed July 30, 2016.

63. Weeks J. Farm Policy. *library.CQPress.com*. 2012. Available at: http://library.cqpress.com/cqresearcher/document.php?id=cqresrre2012081000. Accessed August 26, 2015.

64. Harvest Public Media. Lobbyists of all kinds flock to Farm Bill. *HarvestPublicMedia.org*. 2014. Available at: http://harvestpublicmedia.org/article/lobbyists-all-kinds-flock-farm-bill.

65. Matz ML. Agriculture Trumped in the Primaries. *Ofwlaw.com*. 2016. Available at: http://www.ofwlaw.com/2016/01/06/agriculture-trumped-in-the-primaries/.

66. The Pew Charitable Trusts. *Fixing the Oversight of Chemicals Added to Our Food: Findings and Recommendations of Pew's Assessments of the U.S. Food Additives Program*. 2013. Available at: http://www.pewtrusts.org/en/research-and-analysis/reports/2013/11/07/fixing-the-oversight-of-chemicals-added-to-our-food.

# Chapter 6:

1. Weise E. Experts who decide on food additives conflicted. *USA Today*. 2013. Available at: http://www.usatoday.com/story/news/nation/2013/08/07/food-additives-conflict-of-interest/2625211/.

2. Environmental Working Group. EWG's Dirty Dozen Guide to Food Additives: Generally Recognized As Safe-But Is It? *www.ewg.org*. 2014.

Available at: http://www.ewg.org/research/ewg-s-dirty-dozen-guide-food-additives/generally-recognized-as-safe-but-is-it.

3. The Pew Charitable Trusts. *Fixing the Oversight of Chemicals Added to Our Food: Findings and Recommendations of Pew's Assessments of the U.S. Food Additives Program.* 2013. Available at: http://www.pewtrusts.org/en/research-and-analysis/reports/2013/11/07/fixing-the-oversight-of-chemicals-added-to-our-food.

4. Poti JM, Mendez MA, Wen Ng S, Popkin BM. Is the degree of food processing and convenience linked with the nutritional quality of foods purchased by US households? *American Journal of Clinical Nutrition.* 2015;101(6). Available at: http://doi.org/10.3945/ajcn.114.100925.

5. Goldschmidt V. 12 Dangerous And Hidden Food Ingredients In Seemingly Healthy Foods. *www.saveourbones.com.* 2016. Available at: https://saveourbones.com/12-dangerous-ingredients/. Accessed November 12, 2016.

6. Oikawa S, Nishino K, Inoue S, Mizutani T, Kawanishi S. Oxidative DNA damage and apoptosis induced by metabolites of butylated hydroxytoluene. *Biochem PHarmacol.* 1998;56(3):361–370. Available at: https://www.ncbi.nlm.nih.gov/pubmed/9744574.

7. Bauer K, Dwyer-Nield L, Keil K, Koski K, Malkinson A. Butylated hydroxytoluene (BHT) induction of pulmonary inflammation: a role in tumor promotion. *Exp Lung Res.* 2001;27(3):197–216. Available at: https://www.ncbi.nlm.nih.gov/pubmed/11293324.

8. Bauer A, Dwyer-Nield L, Hankin J, Murphy R, Malkinson A. The lung tumor promoter, butylated hydroxytoluene (BHT), causes chronic inflammation in promotion-sensitive BALB/cByJ mice but not in promotion-resistant CXB4 mice. *Toxicology.* 2001;169(1):1–15. Available at: https://www.ncbi.nlm.nih.gov/pubmed/11696405.

9. Sasaki YF, Kawaguchi S, Kamaya A, et al. The comet assay with 8 mouse organs: Results with 39 currently used food additives. *Mutation Research—Genetic Toxicology and Environmental Mutagenesis.* 2002;519(1-2):103–119.

10. Hamishehkar H, Khani S, Kashanian S, Ezzati Nazhad D, Eskandani M. Geno- and cytotoxicity of propyl gallate food additive. *Drug & Chemical Toxicology.* 2014;37(3):241–6. Available at: https://www.ncbi.nlm.nih.gov/pubmed/24160552.

11. Han Y, Moon H, You B, Park W. Propyl gallate inhibits the growth of calf pulmonary arterial endothelial cells via glutathione depletion. *Toxicol in Vitro.* 2010;24(4):1183–9. Available at: https://www.ncbi.nlm.nih.gov/pubmed/20159035.

12. Foti C, Bonamonte D, Cassano N, Conserva A, Vena G. Allergic contact dermatitis to propyl gallate and pentylene glycol in an emollient cream. *Australas J Dermatol.* 2010;51(2):147–8. Available at: https://www.ncbi.nlm.nih.gov/pubmed/20546226.

13. Pandhi D, Vij A, Singal A. Contact depigmentation induced by propyl gallate. *Clin Exp Dematol.* 2011;36(4):366–8. Available at: https://www.ncbi.nlm.nih.gov/pubmed/21564173.

14. Eler G, Peralta R, Bracht A. The action of n-propyl gallate on gluconeogenesis and oxygen uptake in the rat liver. *Chem Biol Interact.* 2009;181(3):390–9. Available at: https://www.ncbi.nlm.nih.gov/pubmed/19616523.

15. Routledge E, Parker J, Odum J, Ashby J, Sumpter J. Some alkyl hydroxy benzoate preservatives (parabens) are estrogenic. *Toxicol Appl PHarmacol.* 1998;153(1):12–9. Available at: https://www.ncbi.nlm.nih.gov/pubmed/9875295.

16. Darbre P, Aljarrah A, Miller W, et al. Concentrations of parabens in human breast tumours. *J Appl Toxicol.* 2004;24(1):5–13. Available at: https://www.ncbi.nlm.nih.gov/pubmed/14745841.

17. Barr L, Metaxan G, Harbach C, Savoy L, Darbre P. Measurement of paraben concentrations in human breast tissue at serial locations across the breast from axilla to sternum. *J Appl Toxicol.* 2012;32(3):219–32. Available at: https://www.ncbi.nlm.nih.gov/pubmed/22237600.

18. Government Accountability Office. *FOOD SAFETY: FDA Should Strengthen Its Oversight of Food Ingredients Determined to Be Generally Recognized as Safe (GRAS).* 2010:74.

19. Curtis N. Harmful if swallowed-The dangers of food irradiation. *www.naturalnews.com.* 2013. Available at: http://www.naturalnews.com/041878_food_irradiation_harmful_nutrition.html.

20. Neltner TG, Kulkarni NR, Alger HM, et al. Navigating the U.S. Food Additive Regulatory Program. *Wiley Online Library.* 2011. Available at: http://onlinelibrary.wiley.com/doi/10.1111/j.1541-4337.2011.00166.x/full. Accessed August 13, 2016.

21. United States Food and Drug Administration. Food Irradiation: What You Need to Know. *www.fda.gov.* 2016. Available at: http://www.fda.gov/Food/ResourcesForYou/Consumers/ucm261680.htm. Accessed August 19, 2016.

22. U.S. House of Representatives. *Food Additives Amendment of 1958.* U.S. House of Representatives; 1958:1784–1789.

23. Neltner T, Maffini M. Generally Recognized as Secret: Chemicals Added to Food in the United States. *Natural Resources Defense Council.* 2014. Available at: https://www.nrdc.org/sites/default/files/safety-loophole-for-chemicals-in-food-report.pdf.

24. Michael Farris. Personal Communication.

25. U.S. Department of Health and Human Services Food and Drug Administration Center for Food Safety and Applied Nutrition. *Guidance for Industry: Considerations Regarding Substances Added to Foods, Including Beverages and Dietary Supplements.*

2014:5. Available at: http://www.fda.gov/downloads/Food/
GuidanceRegulation/GuidanceDocumentsRegulatoryInformation/
IngredientsAdditivesGRASPackaging/UCM381316.pdf.

26. Anon. Generally Recognized as Safe (GRAS). *U.S. Food and Drug
Administration Website*. 2015. Available at: http://www.fda.gov/Food/
IngredientsPackagingLabeling/GRAS/default.htm. Accessed July 7, 2015.

27. National Archives. Guide to the Records of the U.S. House of
Representatives at the National Archives, 1789-1989 (Record Group
233). *www.archives.gov*. 1989. Available at: http://www.archives.gov/
legislative/guide/house/chapter-22-select-food-and-cosmetics.html.
Accessed August 21, 2016.

28. FDA. Significant Dates in U.S. Food and Drug Law History. *FDA*.

29. American Heart Association. Trans Fats. *www.heart.org*. 2015. Available
at: http://www.heart.org/HEARTORG/HealthyLiving/HealthyEating/
Nutrition/Trans-Fats_UCM_301120_Article.jsp#.V7XzFDf7blI.
Accessed August 18, 2016.

30. United States Food and Drug Administration Department of. *Final
Determination Regarding Partially Hydrogenated Oils*. 2015. Available at:
https://s3.amazonaws.com/public-inspection.federalregister.gov/2015-
14883.pdf.

31. Fitzgerald R. *The Hundred-Year Lie: How Food and Medicine Are
Destroying Your Health*. New York, NY: Penguin Group; 2006.

32. Winters D. The FDA's Determination On Artificial Trans Fat: A Long
Time Coming. *healthaffairs.org*. 2015. Available at: http://healthaffairs.
org/blog/2015/06/23/the-fdas-determination-on-artificial-trans-fat-a-
long-time-coming/.

33. United States Food and Drug Administration. FDA Cuts Trans Fat in
Processed Foods. *www.fda.gov*. 2015. Available at: http://www.fda.gov/
ForConsumers/ConsumerUpdates/ucm372915.htm. Accessed August
18, 2016.

34. Morris S. Personal Communication with Steve D. Morris, Director-
Food Safety and Agriculture. 2016.

35. Sciammacco S. Analysis Finds Hormone Disruptor Used in Cosmetics
In Nearly 50 Different Foods. *www.ewg.org*. 2015. Available at: http://
www.ewg.org/release/analysis-finds-hormone-disruptor-used-cosmetics-
nearly-50-different-foods. Accessed August 19, 2016.

36. Feingold.org. Some Studies on BHT, BHA & TBHQ. *www.feingold.org*.
2012. Available at: http://www.feingold.org/Research/bht.php.

37. Feingold B. Dietary Management of Juvenile Delinquency. *International
Journal of Offender Therapy and Comparative Criminology*. 1979;23(1).
Available at: http://www.feingold.org/Research/PDFstudies/Feingold-
delinq79.pdf.

38. Stokes J, Scudder C. The effect of butylated hydroxyanisole and butylated hydroxytoluene on behavioral development of mice. *Dev Psychobiol*. 1974;7(4):343–50.

39. U.S. Department of Health and Human Services. *Report on Carcinogens, Butylated Hydroxyanisole*. 2014. Available at: https://ntp.niehs.nih.gov/ntp/roc/content/profiles/butylatedhydroxyanisole.pdf.

40. General Mills. BHT statement. *www.generalmills.com*. 2015. Available at: http://www.generalmills.com/en/News/Issues/BHT-statement. Accessed November 12, 2016.

41. Seaman A. Industry influence found in food additive report. *Reuters Health*. 2013. Available at: http://www.reuters.com/article/us-influence-food-additive-idUSBRE9760MZ20130807.

42. Benson J. Reading food labels more important than ever after FDA admits it isn't doing its job. *Natural News*. 2015. Available at: http://www.naturalnews.com/048352_FDA_labels_food_industry.html.

43. Chassaing, Benoit et al. Dietary emulsifiers impact the mouse gut microbiota promoting colitis and metabolic syndrome. *Nature*. 2015;519.

44. Lerner A, Matthias T. Changes in intestinal tight junction permeability associated with industrial food additives explain the rise in incidence of autoimmune disease. *Autoimmunity Reviews*. 2015;14(6):479–489.

45. Feller S. Food additive may be cause of many allergies, researchers say. *www.upi.com*. 2016. Available at: http://www.upi.com/Health_News/2016/07/14/Food-additive-may-be-cause-of-many-allergies-researchers-say/4591468513168/.

46. Campbell A. Autoimmunity and the Gut. *Autoimmune Diseases*. 2014;152428. Available at: http://doi.org/10.1155/2014/152428.

47. Che J. Campbell Soup Will Cut Artificial Ingredients From Its Foods. *www.huffingtonpost.com*. 2015. Available at: http://www.huffingtonpost.com/entry/campbell-soup-artificial-ingredients_us_55b15a5ee4b0224d8831945e.

48. Kaplan J. Campbell to Cut Artificial Flavors, Colors by End of 2018. *www.bloomberg.com*. 2015. Available at: http://www.bloomberg.com/news/articles/2015-07-22/campbell-soup-to-cut-artificial-flavors-colors-by-end-of-2018.

49. Sewalt VP. *GRAS Notification-Exemption Claim*. Palo Alto; 2015. Available at: http://www.fda.gov/downloads/Food/IngredientsPackagingLabeling/GRAS/NoticeInventory/UCM441510.

50. Keefe D. Agency Response Letter GRAS Notice No. GRN 000567. *U.S. Food and Drug Administration Website*. 2015. Available at: http://www.fda.gov/Food/IngredientsPackagingLabeling/GRAS/NoticeInventory/ucm449888.htm. Accessed July 8, 2015.

51. Benson J. "Safety assessments" on nearly all common food additives found to be manipulated by processed food industry: Study. *Natural*

*News*. 2013. Available at: http://www.naturalnews.com/041703_safety_ assessments_food_additives_processed_industry.html.

52. Giammona C. Papa John's Is Spending $100 Million a Year to Clean Up Menu. *www.bloomberg.com*. 2015. Available at: http://www.bloomberg. com/news/articles/2015-06-23/papa-john-s-is-spending-100-million-a-year-to-clean-up-its-menu.

53. Anon. History of the GRAS List and SCOGS Reviews. *U.S. Food and Drug Administration Website*. 2013. Available at: http://www.fda.gov/ Food/IngredientsPackagingLabeling/GRAS/SCOGS/ucm084142.htm. Accessed July 7, 2015.

54. Gaynor, Paulette PD. How U.S. FDA's GRAS Notification Program Works. *www.fda.gov*. Available at: http://www.fda.gov/Food/ IngredientsPackagingLabeling/GRAS/ucm083022.htm. Accessed June 19, 2016.

55. Nicole W. Secret Ingredients: Who Knows What's in Your Food? *Environmental Health Perspectives*. 2013. Available at: http://ehp.niehs. nih.gov/121-a126/. Accessed August 13, 2016.

56. United States Food and Drug Administration Department. Substances Generally Recognized as Safe; Docket No. FDA-1997-N-0020 (formerly 97N-0103). *Federal Register*. 2016;81(159). Available at: https://www.regulations.gov/document?D=FDA-1997-N-0020-0126.

57. Oaklander M. The Soy Milk Ingredient That's Getting the Axe. *time.com*. 2014. Available at: http://time.com/3162074/carrageenan-whitewave/.

58. Food Babe. Breaking: Major Company Removing Controversial Ingredient Carrageenan Because of You! *foodbabe.com*. 2014. Available at: http://foodbabe.com/2014/08/19/breaking-major-company-removing-controversial-ingredient-carrageenan-because-of-you/ comment-page-4/.

59. International Agency for Research on Cancer. *Alcohol drinking*. 1998. Available at: https://web.archive.org/web/20070927120656/http:// monographs.iarc.fr/ENG/Monographs/vol44/volume44.pdf.

60. Andrews D. Synthetic ingredients in Natural Flavors and Natural Flavors in Artificial flavors. *www.ewg.org*. Available at: http://www.ewg. org/foodscores/content/natural-vs-artificial-flavors.

61. Hallagan JB, Hall RL. FEMA GRAS- A GRAS Assessment Program for Flavor Ingredients. *Regulatory Toxicology and Pharmacology*. 1995;21(3):422–430.

62. National Toxicology Program. *Toxicology and Carcinogenesis Studies of Isoeugenol*. Research Triangle Park; 2010. Available at: https://ntp.niehs. nih.gov/ntp/htdocs/lt_rpts/tr551.pdf.

63. R.L. SMITH, W.J. WADDELL, S.M. COHEN, V.J. FERON, L.J. MARNETT, P.S. PORTOGHESE, I.M.C.M. RIETJENS, T.B. ADAMS, C. LUCAS GAVIN, M.M. MCGOWEN, S.V.

TAYLOR and MCW. *GRAS Flavoring Substances 24*. 2009. Available at: http://www.ift.org/knowledge-center/focus-areas/product-development-and-ingredient-innovations/~/media/Food Technology/pdf/2009/06/0609feat_GRAS24text.pdf.

64. Hunt K. A big commitment for Big G cereal. *www.blog.generalmills.com*. 2015. Available at: http://blog.generalmills.com/2015/06/a-big-commitment-for-big-g-cereal/.

65. U.S. Food and Drug Administration. GRAS Notice Inventory, GRN No. 225 and NRDC, Main FDA Response to FOIA. 2014:197.

66. Anon. Theobromine. *VIAS Encyclopedia*. 2005. Available at: http://www.vias.org/encyclopedia/orgchem_theobromine.html. Accessed June 19, 2016.

67. Mike Adams. Personal Communication. 2016.

68. U.S. Food and Drug Administration. *Preliminary Regulatory Impact Analysis for the Proposed Rules for Current Good Manufacturing Practices and Hazard Analysis and Risk-Based Preventive Controls for Human Food, Docket No. FDA-2011-N-0920*. 2013. Available at: http://www.fda.gov/downloads/Food/GuidanceRegulation/FSMA/UCM334117.pdf

69. Kraft. ICONIC KRAFT MACARONI & CHEESE TO REMOVE SYNTHETIC COLORS AND ARTIFICIAL PRESERVATIVES IN THE U.S. IN 2016. *www.newscenter.kraftfoodsgroup.com*. 2015. Available at: http://newscenter.kraftfoodsgroup.com/phoenix.zhtml?c=253200&p=irol-newsArticle&ID=2037718. Accessed November 12, 2016.

70. Kraft. FAQ. *www.kraftmacandcheese.com*. 2015. Available at: http://www.kraftmacandcheese.com/faq. Accessed November 12, 2016.

71. Wonder. Wonder White Bread 570 g. *Wonder Bread*. Available at: http://www.wonderbread.ca. Accessed July 12, 2015.

## Chapter 7:

1. Robbins J. Female Infants Growing Breasts: Another Disaster From Hormones in Milk Production. *Huffington Post*. 2010. Available at: http://www.huffingtonpost.com/john-robbins/female-infants-growing-br_b_676402.html. Accessed May 5, 2015.

2. Pines A, Rozen P, Ron E, Gilat T. Gastrointestinal tumors in acromegalic patients. *The American journal of gastroenterology*. 1985;80(4):266–269.

3. Orme SM, McNally RJQ, Cartwright RA, Belchetz PE. Mortality and Cancer Incidence in Acromegaly: A Retrospective Cohort Study. *Journal of clinical endocinology and metabolism*. 1998;83(8):2730–2734.

4. Epstein S. Unlabeled milk from cows treated with biosynthetic growth hormones: a case of regulatory abdication. *International Journal of Health Services*. 1996;261:173–185.

5.  Manousos O, Souglakos J, Bosetti C, et al. IGF-I and IGF-II in relation to colorectal cancer. *International Journal of Cancer*. 1999;83(1):15–17.

6.  Ma J, Pollak MN, Giovannucci E, et al. Prospective study of colorectal cancer risk in men and plasma levels of insulin-like growth factor (IGF)-I and IGF-binding protein-3. *J Natl Cancer Inst*. 1999;91(7):620–625. Available at: http://www.ncbi.nlm.nih.gov/ entrez/query.fcgi?cmd=Retrieve&db=PubMed&dopt=Citation&list_ uids=10203281.

7.  Giovannucci E, Pollak MN, Platz EA, et al. A prospective study of plasma insulin-like growth factor-1 and binding protein-3 and risk of colorectal neoplasia in women. *Cancer Epidemiol Biomarkers Prev*. 2000;9(4):345–349. Available at: http://www.ncbi.nlm.nih.gov/ entrez/query.fcgi?cmd=Retrieve&db=PubMed&dopt=Citation&list_ uids=10794477.

8.  Renehan AG, Painter JE, O'Halloran D, et al. Circulating insulin-like growth factor II and colorectal adenomas. *J Clin Endocrinol Metab*. 2000;85(9):3402–3408.

9.  Rinaldi S, Cleveland R, Norat T, et al. Serum levels of IGF-I, IGFBP-3 and colorectal cancer risk: Results from the EPIC cohort, plus a meta-analysis of prospective studies. *International Journal of Cancer*. 2010;126(7):1702–1715.

10. Juul A et al. The ratio between serum levels of IGF-1 and the IGF binding protein decreases with age in healthy patients and is increased in acromegalic patients. *Clinical Endocrinology*. 1994;41(85-93).

11. Cascinu S, Del Ferro E, Grianti C, et al. Inhibition of tumor cell kinetics and serum insulin growth factor I levels by octreotide in colorectal cancer patients. *Gastroenterology*. 1997;113(3):767–72. Available at: https://www.ncbi.nlm.nih.gov/pubmed/9287967.

12. Furlanetto RW, DiCarlo JN. Somatomedin-C receptors and growth effects in human breast cells maintained in long-term tissue culture. *Cancer Research*. 1984;44(5):2122–2128.

13. Epstein S. Role of the insulin-like growth factors in cancer development and progression. *Journal of the National Cancer Institute*. 2001;93(3):238.

14. Yu, H; Rohan T. Role of the insulin-like growth factor family in cancer development and progression. *Journal of the National Cancer Institute*. 2000;92:1472–1484.

15. Toniolo P et al. Serum insulin-like growth factor-1 and breast cancer. *International Journal of Cancer*. 2000;88(5):828–832.

16. Agurs-Collins T et al. Insulin-like growth factor-1 and breast cancer risk in post-menopausal American women. *Proceedings of the American Association of Cancer Research 40*. 1999:152.

17.  Hankinson S et al. Circulating concentrations of insulin-like growth factor-1 and risk of breast cancer. *The Lancet.* 1998;351:1393–1396.

18.  Del Giudice ME, Fantus IG, Ezzat S, et al. Insulin and related factors in premenopausal breast cancer risk. *Breast Cancer Res.Treat.* 1998;47(2):111–120.

19.  Bohlke K et al. Insulin-like growth factor-1 in relation to premenopausal ductal carcinoma in situ of the breast. *Epidemiology.* 1998;9(5):570–573.

20.  LeRoith D. Insulin-like growth factors and cancer. *Annals of Internal Medicine.* 1995;122(1):54–59.

21.  Bruning P et al. Insulin-like growth factor-binding protein 3 is decreased in early-stage operable pre-menopausal breast cancer. *International Journal of Cancer.* 1995;62(3):266–270.

22.  Pappa V et al. Insulin-like growth factor-1 receptors are over expressed and predict a low risk in human breast cancer. *Cancer Research.* 1993;53:3736–3740.

23.  Lippman M. The development of biological therapies for breast cancer. *Science.* 1993;259(631-632).

24.  Pollak M et al. Tamoxifen reduced inisulin-like growth factor-1 (IGF-1). *Breast Cancer Research Treatment 22 (Suppl).* 1992:91–100.

25.  Harris J et al. Breast Cancer. *New England Journal of Medicine.* 1992;7:473–480.

26.  Rosen N et al. Insulin-like growth factors in human breast cancer. In: *Breast Cancer Research Treatment 18 (Suppl).*; 1991:555–562.

27.  Lippman A. Growth factors, receptors and breast cancer. *National Institutes of Health Research.* 1991;3:59–62.

28.  Reynolds RK, Talavera F, Roberts JA, Hopkins MP, Menon KM. Regulation of epidermal growth factor and insulin-like growth factor I receptors by estradiol and progesterone in normal and neoplastic endometrial cell cultures. *Gynecologic oncology.* 1990;38(3):396–406.

29.  Glimm DR, Baracos VE, Kennelly JJ. Effect of bovine somatotropin on the distribution of immunoreactive insulin-like growth factor-I in lactating bovine mammary tissue. *Journal of dairy science.* 1988;71(11):2923–2935.

30.  Stoll BA. Breast cancer: further metabolic-endocrine risk markers? *British Journal of Cancer.* 1997;76(12):1652–1654. Available at: https://www.ncbi.nlm.nih.gov/pmc/articles/PMC2228209/.

31.  Badr M, Hassan T, Tarhony S, Metwally W. Insulin-like growth factor-1 and childhood cancer risk. *Oncol Lett.* 2010;1(6):1055–1059. Available at: http://www.ncbi.nlm.nih.gov/pmc/articles/PMC3412533/.

32.  Ross J, Perentesis J, Robison L, Davies S. Big babies and infant leukemia: a role for insulin-like growth factor-1? *Cancer Causes Control.* 1996;7(5):553–559.

33. Wolk A, Mantzoros CS, Andersson SO, et al. Insulin-like growth factor 1 and prostate cancer risk: a population-based, case-control study. *J Natl Cancer Inst.* 1998;90(0027-8874):911–915.

34. Roddam AW, Allen NE, Appleby P, et al. Insulin-like growth factors, their binding proteins, and prostate cancer risk: Analysis of individual patient data from 12 prospective studies. *Annals of Internal Medicine.* 2008;149(7):461–471.

35. Chan JM. Plasma Insulin-Like Growth Factor-I and Prostate Cancer Risk: A Prospective Study. *Science.* 1998;279(5350):563–566.

36. Stattin P, Bylund A, Rinaldi S, et al. Plasma insulin-like growth factor-I, insulin-like growth factor-binding proteins, and prostate cancer risk: a prospective study. *J Natl Cancer Inst.* 2000;92(0027-8874):1910–1917.

37. Stattin P, Rinaldi S, Biessy C, et al. High levels of circulating insulin-like growth factor-I increase prostate cancer risk: A prospective study in a population-based nonscreened cohort. *Journal of Clinical Oncology.* 2004;22(15):3104–3112.

38. Cohen P, Peehl DM, Lamson G, Rosenfeld RG. Insulin-like growth factors (IGFs), IGF receptors, and IGF-binding proteins in primary cultures of prostate epithelial cells. *Journal of Clinical Endocrinology and Metabolism.* 1991;73(2):401–407.

39. Chan J, Stampfer M, Giovannucci E, et al. Plasma insulin-like growth factor-I and prostate cancer risk: a prospective study. *Science.* 1998;279(5350):563–6. Available at: https://www.ncbi.nlm.nih.gov/pubmed/9438850.

40. Mercola. 10 American Foods that are Banned in Other Countries. *topinfopost.com.* 2013.

41. Gucciardi A. Banned in 27 Countries, Monsanto's RBGH Inhabits Many U.S. Dairy Products. *NaturalSociety.com.* 2011.

42. USDA. Dairy 2007 Part I: Reference of Dairy Cattle Health and Management Practices in the United States, 2007. *Veterinary Services, Animal and Plant Health Inspection Services, U.S. Department of Agriculture.* 2007:79.

43. FoodandWaterWatch.org. *rBGH: Anything but Green.* 2008. Available at: http://www.foodandwaterwatch.org/factsheet/rbgh-anything-but-green/.

44. Poti JM, Mendez MA, Wen Ng S, Popkin BM. Is the degree of food processing and convenience linked with the nutritional quality of foods purchased by US households? *American Journal of Clinical Nutrition.* 2015;101(6). Available at: http://doi.org/10.3945/ajcn.114.100925.

45. GAO. *Recombinant Bovine Growth Hormone: FDA Approval Should Be Withheld Until the Mastitis Issue is Resolved.* 1992:68.

46. Mercola. The Dangers of rBGH in Your Milk. *Care2.com.* 2011.

47. Smith JM. *Seeds of Deception: Exposing Industry and Government Lies About the Safety of the Genetically Engineered Foods You're Eating.* Fairfield, IA: Yes Books; 2003.

48. Smith JM. *Genetic Roulette: The Gamble of Our Lives.* Institute for Responsible Technology [Fairfield, IA]; 2012.

49. Chopra S et al. *rBST (Nutrilac) "GAPS Analysis" Report.* Ottawa; 1998.

50. United States Department of Agriculture NASS. Livestock Slaughter. *www.usda.gov.* 2016.

51. Provincial Health Officer's Annual Report. *Food, Health and Well-Being in British Columbia.* British Columbia Ministry of Health Office of the Provincial Health Officer; 2005.

52. Hallberg M. Historical Perspective on Adjustment in the Food and Agricultural Sector. *Penn State University.* 2003.

53. USDA. *Milk Production, Disposition, and Income: 2014 Summary.* 2015.

54. Epstein, Samuel MD. *What's In Your Milk? An Expose of Industry and Government Cover-Up on the DANGERS of the Genetically Engineered (rBGH) Milk You're Drinking.* Victoria: Trafford Publishing; 2006.

55. Dohoo IR, DesCôteaux L, Leslie K, et al. A meta-analysis review of the effects of recombinant bovine somatotropin. 2. Effects on animal health, reproductive performance, and culling. *Canadian journal of veterinary research = Revue canadienne de recherche vétérinaire.* 2003;67(4):252–64.

56. Cohen R. *Milk: The Deadly Poison.* First. Englewood Cliffs, NJ: Argus Publishing; 1998.

57. Cohen R. PUS Expose: Your State's Average Pus Count. *notmilk.com.* Available at: http://www.notmilk.com/lawbreakers.html. Accessed May 7, 2015.

58. Millstone E et al. Plagiarism or protecting public health? *Nature.* 1994;371:647–648.

59. U.S. Department of Health and Human Services, Public Health Service F and DA. Grade "A" Pasteurized Milk Ordinance. *www.fda.gov.* 2009. Available at: http://www.fda.gov/downloads/Food/GuidanceRegulation/ UCM209789.pdf.

60. Hudson W. CDC: "Nightmare bacteria" spreading. *CNN.com.* 2013. Available at: http://www.cnn.com/2013/03/06/health/super-bug-bacteria-spreading/.

61. Bittman M. *A Bone to Pick: The good and bad news about food, with wisdom and advice on diets, food safety, GMOs, farming and more.* New York: Pam Krauss Books; 2015.

62. Murphy R. *GAO Report regarding alleged conflicts of interest in FDA.* Washington DC\; 1994.

63. FDA. *Consumer Report.* 1988.

64. Hardin P. Personal Communication. 2016.

65. Waters A, Contente-Cuomo T, Jordan B, et al. Multidrug-Resistant Staphylococcus aureus in US Meat and Poultry. *Clin Infect Dis.* 2011;52(10):1227–1230.

66. Velloso CP. Regulation of muscle mass by growth homrone and IGF-1. *British Journal of Pharmacology.* 2008;154(3):557–568.

67. Pollak M. Insulin and insulin-like growth factor signalling in neoplasia. *Nat Rev Cancer.* 2008;8(12):915–928. Available at: http://www.ncbi.nlm.nih.gov/entrez/query.fcgi?cmd=Retrieve&db=PubMed&dopt=Citation&list_uids=19029956.

68. Yu H, Rohan T. Role of the insulin-like growth factor family in cancer development and progression. *Journal of the National Cancer Institute.* 2000;92(18):1472–1489.

69. Daxenberger A, Breier BH, Sauerwein H. Increased milk levels of insulin-like growth factor 1 (IGF-1) for the identification of bovine somatotropin (bST) treated cows. *The Analyst.* 1998;123(12):2429–2435.

70. Kusserow RP. *Audit of Issues Related to the Food and Drug Administration Review of Bovine Somatotropin (A-15-90-00046).* 1992:23.

71. FDA. *Report on the Food and Drug Administration's Review of the Safety of Recombinant Bovine Somatotropin.* 1999.

72. Cohen R. Personal Communication. *Phone Interview.* 2016.

73. Taylor M. Interim Guidance on the Voluntary Labeling of Milk and Milk Products From Cows That Have Not Been Treated With Recombinant Bovine Somatotropin. *Federal Register.* 1994;59(28). Available at: http://www.gpo.gov/fdsys/pkg/FR-1994-02-10/html/94-3214.htm.

74. Stranahan S. Monsanto vs. the Milkman. *Mother Jones.* 2004. Available at: http://www.motherjones.com/politics/2004/01/monsanto-vs-milkman.

75. Mohl B. Monsanto: Hormone claim is deceptive. *Boston Globe.* 2003. Available at: https://www.organicconsumers.org/old_articles/rbgh/oakhurst121603.php. Accessed May 5, 2015.

76. Barboza D. Monsanto Sues Dairy in Main Over Label's Remarks on Hormones. *The New Tork Times.* 2003.

77. Mack S. Maine Dairy Caves In to Pressure from Monsanto on rBGH-Free Labeline. *Organic Consumers Association.* 2003. Available at: https://www.organicconsumers.org/old_articles/monsanto/mainegives122903.php. Accessed May 5, 2015.

78. Smith JM. Obama's Team Includes Dangerous Biotech "Yes Men." *Institute for Responsible Technology.* 2008.

79. Moulton L. Labeling Milk from Cows Not Treated with rBST: Legal in all 50 States as of September 29th, 2010. *stir.org.* 2010. Available at: http://stlr.org/2010/10/28/labeling-milk-from-cows-not-treated-with-rbst-legal-in-all-50-states-as-of-september-29th-2010/. Accessed September 27, 2016.

80. Anon. International Dairy Foods Association; Organic Trade Association v. Robert J. Boggs, in his official capacity as Ohio Director of Agriculture. 2010;Nos. 09-35. Available at: http://www.opn.ca6. uscourts.gov/opinions.pdf/10a0322p-06.pdf.

81. Juskevich, Judith; Guyer G. Bovine growth hormone: human food safety evaluation. *Science*. 1990;249(4971). Available at: http://science. sciencemag.org/content/249/4971/875.long.

82. Juskevich, Judith; Guyer G. Bovine growth hormone: human food safety evaluation. *Science*. 1990;249(4971):875–884.

83. Groenewegen PP, McBride BW, Burton JH, Elsasser TH. Bioactivity of milk from bST-treated cows. *The Journal of nutrition*. 1990;120(5):514– 520.

84. Cohen R. Robert Cohen testimony before FDA panel. Available at: http://www.ecoglobe.org/nz/news1999/d049news.htm.

85. Organic Consumers Association. Racketeering Charges Filed Against Donald Rumsfeld & Monsanto. *www.organicconsumers.org*. 2006. Available at: https://www.organicconsumers.org/news/racketeering-charges-filed-against-donald-rumsfeld-monsanto.

86. Boschma J. Monsanto: Big Guy on the Block When it Comes to Friends in Washington. *www.opensecrets.org*. 2013. Available at: https:// www.opensecrets.org/news/2013/02/monsanto/.

87. Madhusoodanan S. Big Food's Revolving Door. *www.stopcorporateabuse. org*. 2015. Available at: https://www.stopcorporateabuse.org/blog/big-foods-revolving-door.

88. Epstein, Samuel and Hardin P. Confidential Monsanto Research Files Dispute Many bGH Safety Claims. *The Milkweed*. 1990.

89. Canine C. Hear No Evil: In its determination to become a model corporate citizen, is the FDA ignoring potential dangers in the nation's food supply? *Eating Well*. 1991.

90. Epstein, Samuel and Hardin P. Epstein & Hardin Respond. *The Milkweed*. 1990.

91. Conyers J. *Letter to Richard R. Kusserow, Inspector General, Department of Health and Human Services*. 1990.

92. Baxter J. Monsanto Accused of Attempt to Bribe Health Canada for rBGH (Posilac) Approval. *The Ottawa Citizen*. 1998:A1.

93. McIlroy A. Pierre Blais thought it was his duty. *Globe and Mail (Canada)*. 1998.

94. Kamen J. Formula for Disaster. *Penthouse*. 1999.

95. The Institute for Responsible Technology. Your Milk on Drugs-Just Say No 1/2. *youtube.com*. 2008. Available at: https://www.youtube.com/ watch?v=_GpqwZDbMHU. Accessed September 4, 2016.

96. Elanco. Somidobove Sustained Release Injection. *New Animal Drug Application*. 1987;7(7):4608.

97. Seife C. Research Misconduct Identified by the US Food and Drug Administration: Out of Sight, Out of Mind, Out of the Peer-Reviewed Literature. *JAMA Internal Medicine*. 2015;175(4):567–577. Available at: http://archinte.jamanetwork.com/article. aspx?articleid=2109855&resultClick=3.

98. Larivière V, Haustein S, Mongeon P. The Oligopoly of Academic Publishers in the Digital Era. *PLOS One*. 2015. Available at: http:// dx.doi.org/10.1371/journal.pone.0127502.

99. Huff E. Academic oligarchy: Majority of science publishing is controlled by just six companies. *Natural News*. 2015. Available at: http://www.naturalnews.com/050457_science_publishing_academic_ oligarchy_corporate_corruption.html.

100. Anon. GM Hormones in Dairy. *Institute for Responsible Technology*.

101. American Farm Bureau Federation. Home page. *www.fb.org*. 2015. Available at: http://www.fb.org/legislative/fbact/. Accessed November 6, 2016.

102. Off C, Douglas J. Whistleblower criticizes deal allowing milk from hormone treated cows into Canada. *www.cbc. ca/radio/asithappens*. 2015. Available at: http://www.cbc.ca/ radio/asithappens/as-it-happens-friday-edition-1.3286136/ updated-whistleblower-criticizes-deal-allowing-milk-from-hormone-treated-cows-into-canada-1.3286156.

103. Dietetics A of N and. About Us. *www.eatrightpro.org*. 2016. Available at: http://www.eatrightpro.org/resources/about-us. Accessed September 1, 2016.

104. Daughaday W, Barbano D. Bovine somatotropin supplemenation of dairy cows. Is the milk safe? *JAMA*. 1990;264(8):1003–5. Available at: https://www.ncbi.nlm.nih.gov/pubmed/2376871.

105. Milk.procon.org. Historical Timeline: History of Cow's Milk from the Ancient World to the Present. Available at: http://milk.procon.org/view. timeline.php?timelineID=000018. Accessed May 3, 2015.

106. RealCaliforniaMilk.com. What We're All About. *Real California Milk*. Available at: http://www.realcaliforniamilk.com/about-us/. Accessed May 3, 2015.

107. MilkPEP. What is MilkPEP? *www.milkpep.org*. Available at: https:// www.milkpep.org/user?destination=milkpep-news. Accessed December 21, 2016.

108. Johnson L. "Got Milk" campaign a fraud-10 better sources of calcium. *Natural News*. 2013. Available at: http://www.naturalnews. com/039613_got_milk_fraud_calcium.html.

109. Hardin P. Personal Communication. 2016.

110. Swiatek J. Eli Lilly's Acquisition of rBGH: OCA Pledges to Pressure the Drug Giant & "Tarnish Their Image." *www.organicconsumers.org*.

2008. Available at: https://www.organicconsumers.org/news/eli-lillys-acquisition-rbgh-oca-pledges-pressure-drug-giant-tarnish-their-image.

111. Raun AP, Preston RL. History of dietylstilbestrol use in cattle. In: *American Society of Animal Science.*; 2002. Available at: https://www.asas.org/docs/publications/raunhist.pdf?sfvrsn=0.

112. Swan SH, Liu F, Overstreet JW, Brazil C, Skakkebaek NE. Semen quality of fertile US males in relation to their mothers' beef consumption during pregnancy. *Human Reproduction.* 2007;22(6):1497–1502.

113. The Organic Center. Growth Hormones Fed to Beef Cattle Damage Human Health. *Organic Consumers Association.* 2007. Available at: https://www.organicconsumers.org/scientific/growth-hormones-fed-beef-cattle-damage-human-health.

114. Henricks DM, Gray SL, Owenby JJ, Lackey BR. Residues from anabolic preparations after good veterinary practice. *APMIS : acta pathologica, microbiologica, et immunologica Scandinavica.* 2001;109(4):273–283.

115. U.S. Food and Drug Administration. *Preliminary Regulatory Impact Analysis for the Proposed Rules for Current Good Manufacturing Practices and Hazard Analysis and Risk-Based Preventive Controls for Human Food, Docket No. FDA-2011-N-0920.* 2013. Available at: http://www.fda.gov/downloads/Food/GuidanceRegulation/FSMA/UCM334117.pdf

116. Bytes O. Monsanto Finally Forced to Dump RBGH. *www.organicconsumers.org.* 2008. Available at: https://www.organicconsumers.org/bytes/organic-bytes-141-monsanto-defeated-safeguarding-organics-dangerous-cell-phones-more. Accessed September 1, 2016.

117. The Organic & Non-GMO Report. Demand for rBST-free milk surges. *www.non-gmoreport.com.* 2006. Available at: http://www.non-gmoreport.com/articles/nov06/rBST_free_milk.php.

118. Starkman N. Grade "A": Getting rbGH Out of School Milk. *civileats.com.* 2009. Available at: http://civileats.com/2009/03/09/grade-a-for-getting-rbgh-out-of-school-milk/. Accessed September 1, 2016.

## Chapter 8:

1. GMO Free News. Monsanto: A Sustainable Agriculture Company. *www.gmoinfo.blogspot.com.* 2013. Available at: http://gmoinfo.blogspot.com/2013/09/monsanto-sustainable-agriculture-company.html. Accessed September 18, 2016.

2. Grocery Manufacturer Association. GROCERY MANUFACTURERS ASSOCIATION POSITION ON GMOS. *The Facts About GMOs; A Project of The Grocery Manufacturers Association.* Available at: http://factsaboutgmos.org/disclosure-statement?_ga=1.19384190.792219552.1483234931. Accessed December 31, 2016.

3.  Poti JM, Mendez MA, Wen Ng S, Popkin BM. Is the degree of food processing and convenience linked with the nutritional quality of foods purchased by US households? *American Journal of Clinical Nutrition*. 2015;101(6).

4.  Corriher SC. Most Americans Are Eating Genetically Engineered Foods Several Times A Day. *The Health Wyze Report & Fidelity Ministry*. 2009. Available at: http://healthwyze.org/reports/281-most-americans-are-eating-genetically-engineered-foods-several-times-a-day.

5.  U.S. FDA. Statement of Policy-Foods Derived from New Plant Varieties. *Federal Register*. 1992;57(no. 104). Available at: http://www.fda.gov/Food/GuidanceRegulation/GuidanceDocumentsRegulatoryInformation/Biotechnology/ucm096095.htm.

6.  World Health Organization. Frequently asked questions on genetically modified foods. *www.who.int*. Available at: http://www.who.int/foodsafety/areas_work/food-technology/faq-genetically-modified-food/en/. Accessed December 17, 2016.

7.  Commoner B. Unraveling the DNA myth: The spurious foundation of genetic engineering. *Harper's*. 2002.

8.  Yang B, Wang J, Tang B, et al. Characterization of Bioactive Recombinant Human Lysozyme Expressed in Milk of Cloned Transgenic Cattle. *PLOS One*. 2011;6(3).

9.  Gucciardi A. Scientists To Add Spider Genes To Human Genome To Create "Bulletproof Skin." *www.naturalsociety.com*. 2012. Available at: http://naturalsociety.com/scientists-to-add-spider-genes-to-human-genome-to-create-bulletproof-skin/.

10. Li Z, Zeng F, Meng F, et al. Generation of transgenic pigs by cytoplasmic injection of piggyBac transposase-based pmGENIE-3 plasmids. *Biol Reprod*. 2014;90(5):93.

11. Rahman M, Mak R, Ayad H, Smith A, Maclean N. Expression of a novel piscine growth hormone gene results in growth enhancement in transgenic tilapia (Oreochromis niloticus). *Transgenic Res*. 1998;7(5):357–69.

12. Davis N, Rawlinson K. Scientists attempting to harvest human organs in pigs create human-pig embryo. *www.theguardian.com*. 2016. Available at: https://www.theguardian.com/science/2016/jun/05/organ-research-scientists-combine-human-stem-cells-and-pig-dna.

13. U.S. Department of Health and Human Services. Animal & Veterinary Consumer Q&A. *www.fda.gov*. 2015. Available at: http://www.fda.gov/AnimalVeterinary/DevelopmentApprovalProcess/GeneticEngineering/GeneticallyEngineeredAnimals/ucm113672.htm. Accessed September 18, 2016.

14. Cummins R, Lilliston B. *Genetically Engineered Food: A Self-Defense Guide for Consumers*. New York, NY: Marlowe & Company; 2000.

15. Sarjeet S, Cowles E, Pietrantonio P. The Mode of Action of Bacillus Thuringiensis Endotoxins. *Annual Review of Entomology*. 1992;37:615–634.

16. Noteborn HP, Bienenmann-Ploum JM, van den Berg ME, et al. Safety assessment of the Bacillus thuringiensis insecticidal crystal protein CRYIA(b) expressed in transgenic tomatoes. In: Engels KH, Takeoka GR, Teranishi R, eds. *ACS Symposium Series 605 Genetically Modified Foods - Safety Issues; American Chemical Society*. Washington DC; 1995:135–147.

17. Pusztai A, Bardocz B, Ewen SWB. Genetically Modified Foods: Potential Human Health Effects. In: D'Mello JP., ed. *CAB International; Food Safety: Contimainats and Toxins*.; 2003:347–372. Available at: http://www.bioemit.math.ntnu.no/meetings/pusztaibookK.pdf.

18. El-Shamei Z, Gab-Alla A, Shatta A, Moussa E, Rayan A. Histopathological change in some organs of male rats fet on genetically modified corn. *J Am Sci*. 2012;8(10):684–96.

19. Rinamore A, Roselli M, Britti S, et al. Intestinal and peripheral immune response to MON810 maize ingestion in weaning and old mice. *J Agric Food Chem*. 2008;56(23):11533–9.

20. Vázquez-Padrón, RI Gonzáles-Cabrera, J García-Tovar C, Neri-Bazan L, Lopéz-Revilla, R Hernández M, Moreno-Fierro L, de la Riva G. Cry1Ac protoxin from Bacillus thuringiensis sp. kurstaki HD73 binds to surface proteins in the mouse small intestine. *Biochem Biophys Res Commun*. 2000;271(1):54–8.

21. GMO Science. Are all forms of Bt toxin safe? *GMO Science*. 2015. Available at: https://www.gmoscience.org/is-bt-toxin-safe/.

22. United States Department of Agriculture; Economic Research Service. Recent Trends in GE Adoption. *www.ers.usda.gov*. 2016. Available at: https://www.ers.usda.gov/data-products/adoption-of-genetically-engineered-crops-in-the-us/recent-trends-in-ge-adoption.aspx. Accessed December 17, 2016.

23. Johnson D, O'Connor S. These Charts Show Every Genetically Modified Food People Already Eat in the U.S. *Time*. 2015. Available at: http://time.com/3840073/gmo-food-charts/.

24. United States Department of Agriculture Economic Research Service. Sugar & Sweeteners Policy. *usda.gov*. 2015. Available at: http://www.ers.usda.gov/topics/crops/sugar-sweeteners/policy.aspx. Accessed July 20, 2016.

25. Institute for Responsible Technology. FAQs: What's a GMO? *www.responsibletechnology.org*. Available at: http://www.responsibletechnology.org/faqs. Accessed August 18, 2015.

26. Justice Thomas. ASSOCIATION FOR MOLECULAR PATHOLOGY ET AL. v. MYRIAD GENETICS, INC., ET AL. 2013;No. 12-398.

Available at: https://www.supremecourt.gov/opinions/12pdf/12-398_1b7d.pdf.

27. University of California San Diego. Bacillus thuringiensis. *www.bt.ucsd.edu/organic_farming.html*. Available at: http://www.bt.ucsd.edu/organic_farming.html. Accessed November 9, 2016.

28. Pusztai S. Bt in organic farming and GM crops - the difference. *GMWatch.org*. 2016. Available at: http://www.gmwatch.org/latest-listing/40-2001/1058-bt-in-organic-farming-and-gm-crops-the-difference-. Accessed November 9, 2016.

29. Johal GS, Huber DM. Glyphosate effects on diseases of plants. *European Journal of Agronomy*. 2009;31(3):144–152.

30. Bøhn T, Cuhra M, Traavik T, et al. Compositional differences in soybeans on the market: Glyphosate accumulates in Roundup Ready GM soybeans. *Food Chemistry*. 2014;153:207–215.

31. Lundberg DS, Lebeis SL, Paredes SH, et al. Defining the core Arabidopsis thaliana root microbiome. *Nature*. 2012;488:86–90.

32. Kremer RJ, Means NE. Glyphosate and glyphosate-resistant crop interactions with rhizosphere microorganisms. *European Journal of Agronomy*. 2009;31(3):153–161.

33. Lappe M, Bailey B, Childress C, Setchell K. Alterations in Clinically Important Phytoestrogens in Genetically Modified, Herbicide-Tolerant Soybeans. *Journal of Medicinal Food*. 2009;1(4):241–245.

34. Lissin L, Cooke J. Phytoestrogens and cardiovascular health. *J Am Coll Cardiol*. 2000;35(6):1403–1410. Available at: http://www.ncbi.nlm.nih.gov/pubmed/10807439.

35. Benbrook CM. Impacts of genetically engineered crops on pesticide use in the U.S.—the first sixteen years. *Environmental Sciences Europe*. 2012;24(1):1–13. Available at: http://dx.doi.org/10.1186/2190-4715-24-24.

36. Beville R. How Pervasive are GMOs in Animal Feed? *GMOinside.org*. 2013. Available at: http://gmoinside.org/gmos-in-animal-feed/. Accessed November 7, 2016.

37. United States Department of Agriculture ERS. Corn: Background. *www.ers.usda.gov*. 2016. Available at: https://www.ers.usda.gov/topics/crops/corn/background/. Accessed December 17, 2016.

38. Andhra P. *Mortality in Sheep Flocks after grazing on Bt Cotton fields Warangal District, Andhra Pradesh*. Warangal District; 2006. Available at: http://gmwatch.org/latest-listing/1-news-items/6416-mortality-in-sheep-flocks-after-grazing-on-bt-cotton-fields-warangal-district-andhra-pradesh-2942006.

39. Ho M-W. GM Ban Long Overdue. *ISIS Report*. 2006. Available at: http://www.i-sis.org.uk/GMBanLongOverdue.php. Accessed September 19, 2016.

40. Vecchio L, Cisterna B, Malatesta M, Martin T, Biggiogera M. Ultrastructural analysis of testes from mice fed on genetically modified soybean. *Eur J Histochem*. 2004;48(4):448–54.

41. Al. O et. Temporary Depression of Transcription in Mouse Pre-implantation Embryos from Mice Fed on Genetically Modified Soybeans. In: *48th Symposium of the Society for Histochemistry*. Lake Maggiore (Italy); 2006.

42. Velimirov A, Binter C. Biological effects of transgenic maize NK603 x MON810 fed in long term reproduction studies in mice. In: *Forschungsberichte der Sektion IV.*; 2008.

43. Ermakova I. Experimental Evidence of GMO Hazards. In: *Scientists for a FM Free Europe, EU Parliament*. Brussels; 2007.

44. Ermakova I. Genetically modified organisms and biological risks. In: *Proceedings of International Disaster Reduction Conferences (IDRC)*. Davos, Switzerland; 2006:168–172. Available at: http://www.whale. to/a/genetically.html.

45. Ermakova I. GMO: Life itself intervened into the experiments. *Letter, EcosInform*. 2006;N2:3–4.

46. Ermakova I. Influence of genetically modified soya on the birth-weight and survival of rat pups. In: *Epigenetics, Transgenic Plants & Risk Assessment.*; 2013. Available at: http://somloquesembrem.org/ wp-content/uploads/2013/01/Ermakovasoja.pdf.

47. Malatesta M, Boraldi F, Annovi G, et al. A long-term study on female mice fed on a genetically modified soybean: effects on liver ageing. *Histochem Cell Biol*. 2008;130(5):967–77. Available at: http://www. ncbi.nlm.nih.gov/pubmed/18648843.

48. Pusztai A. Can science give us the tools for recognizing possible health risks of GM food? *Nutr Health*. 2002;16(2):73–84.

49. Lemen J, Hammond B, Riordan S, Jiang C, Nemeth M. *Summary of Study CV-2000-260: 13-Week Dietary Subchronic Comparison Study with MON 863 Corn in Rats Preceded by a 1-Week Baseline Food Consumption Determination with PMI Certified Rodent Diet #5002; Report No. MSL-18175*. St. Louis; 2002. Available at: https://www.greenpeace.de/sites/ www.greenpeace.de/files/Monsanto_Rattenfuetterungsstudie_0.pdf.

50. Tudisco R, Lombardi P, Bovera F, D'Angelo D. Genetically modified soya bean in rabbit feeding: detection of DNA fragments and evaluation of metabolic effects by enzymatic analysis. *Animal Science*. 2006;82(2):193–199.

51. Malatesta M, Caporaioni C, Gavaudan S, et al. Ultrastructural morphometrical and immunocytochemical analyses of hepatocyte nuclei from mice fed on genetically modified soybean. *Cell Struct Funct*. 2002;27(4):173–80. Available at: https://www.ncbi.nlm.nih.gov/ pubmed/12441651.

52. Malatesta M, Biggiogera M, Manuali E, et al. Fine structural analyses of pancreatic acinar cell nuclei from mice fed on genetically modified soybean. *Eur J Histochem.* 2003;47(4):385–8.

53. Malatesta M, Caporaioni C, Rossi L, et al. Ultrastructural analysis of pancreatic acinar cells from mice fed on genetically modified soybean. *J Anat.* 2002;201(5):409–415.

54. Finamore A, Roselli M, Britti S, et al. Intestinal and peripheral immune response to MON810 maize ingestion in weaning and old mice. *J Agric Food Chem.* 2008;56(23):11533–9. Available at: http://www.ncbi.nlm. nih.gov/pubmed/19007233.

55. Fares N, El-Sayed A. Fine structural changes in the ileum of mice fed on delta-endotoxin-treated potatoes and transgenic potatoes. *Nat Toxins.* 1998;6(6):219–33. Available at: http://www.ncbi.nlm.nih.gov/pubmed/ ?term=Fine+Structural+Changes+in+the+Ileum+of+Mice+Fed+on+ Endotoxin+Treated+Potatoes+and+Transgenic+Potatoes.

56. SW E, Pusztai A. Effect of diets containing genetically modified potatoes expressing Galanthus nivalis lectin on rat small intestine. *Lancet.* 1999;354(9187):1353–4. Available at: https://www.ncbi.nlm. nih.gov/pubmed/10533866.

57. Vazquez-Padron R, Moreno-Fierros L, Neri-Bazan L, et al. Characterization of the mucosal and systemic immune response induced by Cry1Ac protein from Bacillus thuringiensis HD 73 in mice. *Braz J Med Biol Res.* 2000;33(2):147–55.

58. Vazquez-Padron R, Moreno-Fierros L, Neri-Bazan L, de-la Riva G, Lopez-Revilla R. Bacillus thuringiensis Cry1Ac protoxin is a potent systemic and mucosal adjuvant. *Scand J Immunol.* 1999;49(6):578–84. Available at: http://www.ncbi.nlm.nih.gov/pubmed/?term=Bacillus+ thuringiensis+Cry1Ac+protoxin+is+a+potent+systemic+and+mucosal+ adjuvant.

59. Kroghsbo S, Madsen C, Poulsen M, et al. Immunotoxicological studies of genetically modified rice expressing PHA-E lectin or Bt toxin in Wistar rats. *Toxicology.* 2008;245(1-2):24–34.

60. Dean A, Armstrong J. Genetically Modified Foods. *www.aaemonline. org.* 2009. Available at: http://www.aaemonline.org/gmo.php. Accessed September 15, 2016.

61. Smith JM. *Seeds of Deception: Exposing Industry and Government Lies About the Safety of the Genetically Engineered Foods You're Eating.* Fairfield, IA: Yes Books; 2003.

62. Samsel A, Seneff S. Glyphosate's Suppression of Cytochrome P450 Enzymes and Amino Acid Biosynthesis by the Gut Microbiome: Pathways to Modern Diseases. *Entropy.* 2013;15(4):1416–1463. Available at: http://www.mdpi.com/1099-4300/15/4/1416.

63. Thongprakaisang S, Thiantanawat A, Rangkadilok N, Suriyo T, Satayavivad J. Glyphosate induces human breast cancer cells growth via estrogen receptors. *Food Chem. Toxicol.* 2013;59:129–36. Available at: http://www.ncbi.nlm.nih.gov/pubmed/23756170.

64. Benachour N, Séralini GE. Glyphosate formulations induce apoptosis and necrosis in human umbilical, embryonic, and placental cells. *Chemical Research in Toxicology.* 2009;22(1):97–105.

65. International Agency for Research on Cancer. *IARC Monographs Volume 112: evaluation of five organophosphate insecticides and herbicides.* 2015:2. Available at: http://www.iarc.fr/en/media-centre/iarcnews/pdf/MonographVolume112.pdf.

66. Yum H-Y, Lee S-Y, Lee K-E, Sohn M-H, Kim K-E. Genetically modified and wild soybeans: An immunologic comparison. *Allergy and Asthma Proceedings.* 2005;26(3):210–216(7). Available at: http://www.ingentaconnect.com/content/ocean/aap/2005/00000026/00000003/art00010.

67. Nordlee J, Taylor S, Townsend J, Thomas L, Bush R. Identification of a Brazil-Nut Allergen in Transgenic Soybeans. *The New Englad Journal of Medicine.* 1996;334:688–692. Available at: http://www.nejm.org/doi/full/10.1056/NEJM199603143341103#t=article.

68. Hardell, L and Erickson M. A Case-Controlled Study of non-Hodgkin's Lymphoma and Exposure to Pesticides. *Cancer.* 1999;86(6).

69. Fernandez-Cornejo J, Nehring R, Osteen C, et al. *Pesticide Use in U.S. Agriculture: 21 Selected Crops, 1960-2008.* Washington DC; 2014. Available at: https://www.ers.usda.gov/webdocs/publications/eib124/46734_eib124.pdf.

70. Goldburg R. FDA public hearing on genetically engineered foods.

71. Blewett TC. *Comments on behalf of Dow AgroSciences LLC on Supplemental information for petition for determination of nonregulated status for herbicide resistant DAS-40278-9 Corn. Economic and agronomic impacts of the introduction of DAS-40278-9 corn on glyphosate res.* 2011.

72. Neuman W, Pollack A. Farmers Cope With Roundup-Resistant Weeds. *The New York Times.* 2010. Available at: http://www.nytimes.com/2010/05/04/business/energy-environment/04weed.html?pagewanted=all&_r=0.

73. Rosenboro K. Why Is Glyphosate Sprayed on Crops Right Before Harvest? *Ecowatch.com.* 2016. Available at: http://www.ecowatch.com/why-is-glyphosate-sprayed-on-crops-right-before-harvest-1882187755.html.

74. Main D. Glypohsate Now the Most-Used Agricultural Chemical Ever. *www.newsweek.com.* 2016. Available at: http://www.newsweek.com/glyphosate-now-most-used-agricultural-chemical-ever-422419.

75. Deike J. Monsanto's Roundup Found in 75% of Air and Rain Samples. *www.ecowatch.com*. 2014. Available at: http://www.ecowatch.com/ monsantos-roundup-found-in-75-of-air-and-rain-samples-1881869607. html. Accessed September 16, 2015.

76. Clair E, Mesnage R, Travert C, Séralini G-É. A glyphosate-based herbicide induces necrosis and apoptosis in mature rat testicular cells in vitro, and testosterone decrease at lower levels. *Toxicology in vitro : an international journal published in association with BIBRA*. 2012;26(2):269–79. Available at: http://www.ncbi.nlm.nih.gov/ pubmed/22200534. Accessed October 25, 2012.

77. Vecchio L, Cisterna B, Malatesta M, Martin T, Biggiogera M. Ultrastructural analysis of testes from mice fed on genetically modified soybean . *European Journal of Histochemistry*. 2004. Available at: http://apps.webofknowledge.com. ezproxy.fgcu.edu/full_record.do?product=UA&search_ mode=GeneralSearch&qid=13&SID=2Dipkije2e@ L8hHLALi&page=1&doc=1. Accessed October 25, 2012.

78. Earth Open Source. Truth: So-called "safe" levels of Roundup may not be safe after all. *www.earthopensource.org*. 2015. Available at: http://earthopensource.org/gmomythsandtruths/ sample-page/4-health-hazards-roundup-glyphosate/4-2-myth-strict-regulations-ensure-exposed-safe-levels-roundup/. Accessed September 18, 2016.

79. Bohn T, Cuhra M. How "Extreme Levels" of Roundup in Food Became the Industry Norm. *www.independentsciencenews.org*. 2014. Available at: https://www.independentsciencenews.org/news/how-extreme-levels-of-roundup-in-food-became-the-industry-norm/.

80. Leu A. Monsanto's Toxic Herbicide Glyphosate: A Review of its Health and Environmental Effects. *www.organicconsumers.org*. 2007. Available at: https://www.organicconsumers.org/news/monsantos-toxic-herbicide-glyphosate-review-its-health-and-environmental-effects.

81. Pollan M. *Omnivore's Dilemma: A Natural History of Fourl Meals*. New York: The Penguin Press; 2006.

82. Sharp R. Americans Eat Their Weight In Genetically Engineered Food. *Environmental Working Group*. 2012. Available at: http://www.ewg.org/ agmag/2012/10/americans-eat-their-weight-genetically-engineered-food.

83. Smith JM. *Genetic Roulette: The Gamble of Our Lives*. Institute for Responsible Technology [Fairfield, IA]; 2012.

84. Sarich C. Why Are Government subsidies Forcing GMO Baby Formula on Low Income Mothers? *GlobalResearch*. 2015. Available at: http:// www.globalresearch.ca/why-are-govt-subsidies-forcing-gmo-baby-formula-on-low-income-mothers/5432898.

85. The Detox Project. UCSF Presentation Reveals Glyphosate Contamination in People across America. *www.detoxproject.org.* 2016.

86. Aris A, Leblanc S. Maternal and fetal exposure to pesticides associated to genetically modified foods in Eastern Townships of Quebec, Canada. *Reproductive Toxicology.* 2011;31(4):528–33.

87. Bearer CF. Environmental Health Hazards: How Children Are Different from Adults. *The Future of Children.* 1995;5(2). Available at: https://www.princeton.edu/futureofchildren/publications/docs/05_02_02.pdf.

88. Pesticide Action Network. Children. *www.panna.org.* Available at: http://www.panna.org/human-health-harms/children. Accessed November 8, 2016.

89. Shilhavy B. ALERT: Certified Organic Food Grown in U.S. Found Contaminated with Glyphosate Herbicide. *Health Impact News.* 2014. Available at: http://healthimpactnews.com/2014/alert-certified-organic-food-grown-in-u-s-found-contaminated-with-glyphosate-herbicide/. Accessed November 7, 2016.

90. The Pew Charitable Trusts. *Fixing the Oversight of Chemicals Added to Our Food: Findings and Recommendations of Pew's Assessments of the U.S. Food Additives Program.* 2013. Available at: http://www.pewtrusts.org/en/research-and-analysis/reports/2013/11/07/fixing-the-oversight-of-chemicals-added-to-our-food.

91. Kimbrell A. *Your Right to Know: Genetic Engineering and the Secret Changes in Your Food.* San Rafael: Earth Aware; 2007.

92. GMO Inside. Five Major Food Companies Annouce GMO Labeling. What Should We Expect at the Grocery Store? *www.gmoinside.org.* 2016. Available at: http://gmoinside.org/five-major-food-companies-announce-gmo-labeling-what-should-we-expect-at-the-grocery-store/. Accessed November 9, 2016.

93. U.S. House of Representatives. *Food Additives Amendment of 1958.* U.S. House of Representatives; 1958:1784–1789.

94. Druker S. Why the FDA's Policy on Genetically Engineered Foods Is Irresponsible and Illegal. *www.biointegrity.org.* 2011. Available at: http://www.biointegrity.org/WhyFDAPolicyIrresponsible.htm. Accessed December 8, 2016.

95. Bio-integrity AF. About Steven M. Druker. *www.biointegrity.org.* 1996. Available at: http://www.biointegrity.org/AboutUs.htm. Accessed December 8, 2016.

96. Linda K. *Comments about the Federal Register document "Statement of Policy: Foods from Genetically Modified Plants."* 1992. Available at: www.biointegrity.org.

97. Pribyl LJ. *Comments on the Biotechnology Draft Document, 2/27/92.* 1992. Available at: http://www.biointegrity.org/list.htm.

98. Anon. Document 2 at http://www.biointegrity.org/FDAdocs/index. html.

99. Anon. Document 10 at http://www.biointegrity.org/FDAdocs/index. html.

100. The Lancet. Health risks of genetically modified foods. *The Lancet.* 1999;353(9167):1811. Available at: http://www.thelancet.com/pdfs/ journals/lancet/PIIS0140-6736(99)00093-8.pdf.

101. The Royal Society of Canada. *Elements of Precaution: Recommendations for the Regulation of Food Biotechnology in Canada.* Ottawa; 2001. Available at: http://www.rsc.ca/sites/default/files/pdf/GMreportEN.pdf.

102. Kmietowicz Z. GM foods should be submitted to further studies, says BMA. *British Medical Journal.* 2004;328(7440):602. Available at: https://www.ncbi.nlm.nih.gov/pmc/articles/PMC381159/.

103. Anon. *Public Health Association of Australia: Policy-at-a-glance - Genetically Modified Foods Policy.* Available at: http://www.phaa.net.au/ documents/item/235.

104. Dona A, Arvanitoyannis I. Health risks of genetically modified foods. *Critical Reviews in Food Science and Nutrition.* 2009;49(2):164–75. Available at: https://www.ncbi.nlm.nih.gov/pubmed/18989835.

105. Hilbeck A et al. No scientific consensus of GMO safety. *Environmental Sciences Europe.* 2015;27(4).

106. Alliance For Bio-integrity. About Steven M. Druker. *www. allianceforbiointegrity.com.* Available at: https://allianceforbiointegrity. wordpress.com/about/. Accessed September 16, 2016.

107. Technology I for R. GMO FAQs. *www.responsibletechnology.org.* Available at: http://responsibletechnology.org/gmo-education/faqs/. Accessed September 16, 2016.

108. Marie-Monique R. *The World According to Monsanto: Pollution, Corruption, and the Control of the World's Food Supply.* New York: New Press; 2010.

109. Anon. Document 1 at http://www.biointegrity.org/FDAdocs/index. html.

110. Plume K. USDA confirms unapproved GMO wheat found in Washington state. *Reuters.* 2016. Available at: http://www.reuters.com/ article/us-wheat-washington-gmo-idUSKCN10920K.

111. Phuong L. GMO wheat found in Washington state could affect US trade. *Associated Press.* 2016.

112. Robbins J. Can GMOs Help End World Hunter? *www.huffingtonpost. com.* 2011. Available at: http://www.huffingtonpost.com/john-robbins/ gmo-food_b_914968.html. Accessed September 17, 2016.

113. World Food Programme. What causes hunger? *www.wfp.org.* 2016. Available at: https://www.wfp.org/hunger/causes. Accessed September 18, 2016.

114. Walton RG. *Survey of Aspartame Studies: Correlation of Outcomes and Funding sources.* 1998.

115. Graff G, Cullen S, Bradford K, Zilberman D, Bennett A. The public-private structure of intellectual property ownership in agricultural biotechnology. *Nature Biotechnology.* 2003;21(9). Available at: http://are.berkeley.edu/~zilber11/papers/publicprivate.pdf.

116. Suurkula J. Dysfunctional science: Towards a "pseudoscientific world order?" *Physicians and Scientists for Responsible Application of Science and Technology.* 2000.

117. Druker S. *Altered Genes, Twisted Truth: How the Venture to Genetically Engineer Our Food Has Subverted Science, Corrupted Government, and Systematically Deceived the Public.* Clear River Press; 2015.

118. Smith JM. *Genetic Roulette: The Documented Health Risks of Genetically Engineered Foods.* Fairfield, IA: Yes! Books; 2007.

119. Vidal J. Revolts Against Monsanto and Genetically Engineered Foods throughout Europe. *The Guardian (UK).* 1999.

120. Lambrecht B. *Dinner at the New Gene Cafe: How Genetic Engineering Is Changing What We Eat, How We Live, and the Global Politics of Food.* New York: St. Martin's Press; 2001.

121. Johnson D, O'Connor S. These Charts Show Every Genetically Modified Food People Already Eat in the U.S. *www.time.com.* 2015. Available at: http://time.com/3840073/gmo-food-charts/.

122. Project Censored. Top 25 Archive. *www.projectcensored.org.* 1999. Available at: http://projectcensored.org/top-25-censored-stories-of-all-time/. Accessed September 19, 2016.

123. Consumer Reports. Consumers Want Mandatory Labeling for GMOFoods. *www.consumerreports.org.* 2015. Available at: http://www.consumerreports.org/food-safety/consumers-want-mandatory-labeling-for-gmo-foods/. Accessed November 9, 2016.

124. Just Label It! Labeling Around The World. *www.justlabelit.org.* 2016. Available at: http://www.justlabelit.org/right-to-know-center/labeling-around-the-world/. Accessed November 9, 2016.

125. The Institute for Responsible Technology. Even though Obama just signed the DARK Act... *www.responsibletechnology.org.* 2016. Available at: http://responsibletechnology.org/even-though-obama-just-signed-the-dark-act/. Accessed September 18, 2016.

126. Campbell Team. Why We Support Mandatory National GMO Labeling. *www.campbellsoupcompany.com.* 2016. Available at: https://www.campbellsoupcompany.com/newsroom/news/2016/01/07/labeling/Accessed November 9, 2016.

127. Campbell's. What's In Our Food. *www.whatsinmyfood.com.* 2015. Available at: http://www.whatsinmyfood.com. Accessed November 9, 2016.

128. U.S. Food and Drug Administration. FDA Has Determined That the AquAdvantage Salmon is as Safe to Eat as Non-GE Salmon. *www.fda.gov*. 2015. Available at: http://www.fda.gov/ForConsumers/ConsumerUpdates/ucm472487.htm. Accessed September 15, 2016.

129. United States Department of Agriculture; Animal and Plant Health Inspection Service. Petitions for Determination of Nonregulated Status. *www.aphis.usda.gov*. 2016. Available at: https://www.aphis.usda.gov/aphis/ourfocus/biotechnology/permits-notifications-petitions/petitions/petition-status. Accessed December 31, 2016.

130. Malatesta M, Tiberi C, Baldelli B, et al. Reversibility of hepatocyte nuclear modifications in mice fed on genetically modified soybean. *European Journal of Histochemistry*. 2005;49(3):237–242. Available at: http://www.ncbi.nlm.nih.gov/pubmed/16216809.

131. Ben & Jerry's. Our Non-GMO Standards. *www.benjerry.com*. 2014. Available at: http://www.benjerry.com/values/issues-we-care-about/support-gmo-labeling/our-non-gmo-standards. Accessed September 18, 2016.

132. Cheerios. Cheerios and GMOs: FAQs. *www.cheerios.com*. 2014. Available at: http://www.cheerios.com/en/Articles/cheerios-and-gmos. Accessed September 18, 2016.

133. Turner N, Giammona C. Chipotle Completes Plan to Remove GMOs From Its Menu. *www.bloomberg.com*. 2015. Available at: http://www.bloomberg.com/news/articles/2015-04-27/chipotle-completes-plan-to-remove-gmos-from-all-its-ingredients.

134. Barrett M. Victory: Hershey To Remove GMO Ingredients From Milk Chocolate. *www.naturalsociety.com*. 2015. Available at: http://naturalsociety.com/victory-hershey-remove-gmo-ingredients-milk-chocolate/. Accessed September 19, 2016.

135. Campbell A. Autoimmunity and the Gut. *Autoimmune Diseases*. 2014;152428. Available at: http://doi.org/10.1155/2014/152428.

## Chapter 9:

1. United States Department of Agriculture. Dietary Guidelines For Americans 2015-2020. *www.choosemyplate.gov*. 2016. Available at: https://www.choosemyplate.gov/dietary-guidelines. Accessed September 18, 2016.

2. Teicholz N. The scientific report guiding the US dietary guidelines: is it scientific? *BMJ*. 2015;351. Available at: http://www.bmj.com/content/bmj/351/bmj.h4962.full.pdf.

3. Committee DGA. *Report of the Dietary Guidelines Advisory Committee on the Dietary Guidelines for Americans, 1995*. 1995. Available at: https://health.gov/dietaryguidelines/dga95/pdf/DGREPORT.PDF.

4.   Fan S. The fat-fueled bran: unnatural or advantageous? *www. blogs.scientificamerican.com.* 2013. Available at: https://blogs. scientificamerican.com/mind-guest-blog/the-fat-fueled-brain-unnatural-or-advantageous/. Accessed November 10, 2016.

5.   United States Department of Health and Human Services and United States Department of Agriculture. *Dietary Guidelines for Americans 2015-2020 8th Edition.* Washington DC; 2015. Available at: https:// health.gov/dietaryguidelines/2015/guidelines/.

6.   United States Department of Agriculture. Become a MyPlate Champion. *www.choosemyplate.gov/kids.* 2015. Available at: https:// www.choosemyplate.gov/kids-become-myplate-champion. Accessed November 10, 2016.

7.   United States Department of Agriculture. Teachers. *www.choosemyplate. gov/teachers.* 2016. Available at: https://www.choosemyplate.gov/ teachers. Accessed November 10, 2016.

8.   Teicholz N. *The Big Fat Surprise: Why Butter, Meat & Cheese Belong in a Healthy Diet.* New York, NY: Simon & Schuster Paperbacks; 2014.

9.   American Heart Association. How the Heart-Check Food Certification Program Works. *www.heart.org.* 2016. Available at: http://www.heart.org/HEARTORG/HealthyLiving/HealthyEating/ Heart-CheckMarkCertification/How-the-Heart-Check-Food-Certification-Program-Works_UCM_300133_Article. jsp#.V-UaTDf7bII. Accessed September 23, 2016.

10.  National Heart Lung and Blood Institute. Conquering Cardiovascular Disease. *www.nhlbi.nih.gov.* Available at: https://www.nhlbi.nih.gov/ news/spotlight/success/conquering-cardiovascular-disease. Accessed November 10, 2016.

11.  Keys A. Atherosclerosis: A Problem In Newer Public Health. *Journal of Mt. Sinai Hospital.* 1953;2:134.

12.  Page I, Stare F, Corcoran A, Pollack H, Wilkinson C. Atherosclerosis and the fat content of the diet. *Circulation.* 1957;16(2):163–178.

13.  Page I, Allen E, Chamberlain F, et al. Dietary Fat and Its Relation to Heart Attacks and Strokes. *Circulation.* 1961;23(1):133–136.

14.  Time. Ancel Keys. 1961. Available at: http://content.time.com/time/ covers/0,16641,19610113,00.html. Accessed November 10, 2016.

15.  Keys A. The Seven Countries Study Publications. 2016. Available at: http://www.sevencountriesstudy.com/study-findings/publications/. Accessed November 10, 2016.

16.  Sarri K, Kafatos A. Letter to the Editor: The Seven Countries Study in Crete: olive oil, Mediterranean diet or fasting? *Public Health Nutrition.* 2005;8(6):666.

17.  Sarri K, Linardakis M, Bervanaki F, Tzanakis N, Kafatos A. Greek Orthodox fasting rituals: a hidden characteristic of the Mediterranean diet of Crete. *British Journal of Nutrition.* 2004;92(2):277–84.

18. Keys A, Aravanis C, Sdrin H. The diets of middle-aged men in two rural areas of Greece. *Voeding*. 1966;27:575–586. Available at: https://www.cabdirect.org/cabdirect/abstract/19671404963.

19. Menotti A, Kromhout D, Blackburn H, et al. Food intake patterns and 25-year mortality from coronary heart disease: cross-cultural correlations in the Seven Countries Study. The Seven Countries Study Research Group. *European Journal of Epidemiology*. 1999;15(6):507–15.

20. Torrens K. The truth about low-fat foods. *www.bbcgoodfood.com*. 2016. Available at: http://www.bbcgoodfood.com/howto/guide/truth-about-low-fat-foods. Accessed November 10, 2016.

21. Hyman M. The Fat Summit. In: ; 2016.

22. American Heart Association. The American Heart Association's Diet and Lifestyle Recommendations. 2016. Available at: http://www.heart.org/HEARTORG/HealthyLiving/Diet-and-Lifestyle-Recommendations_UCM_305855_Article.jsp#.V-UZkDf7blI. Accessed September 23, 2016.

23. Crisco. Crisco Our Heritage. *www.crisco.com*. 2016. Available at: http://www.crisco.com/our-heritage. Accessed November 10, 2016.

24. Blasbalg T, Hibbeln J, Ramsden C, Majchrzak S, Rawlings R. Changes in consumption of omega-3 and omega-6 fatty acids in the United States during the 20th century. *American Journal of Clinical Nutrition*. 2011;93(5):950–62. Available at: https://www.ncbi.nlm.nih.gov/pubmed/21367944.

25. United States Food and Drug Administration; Department of Health and Human Services. Final Determination Regarding Partially Hydrogenated Oils; Docket No. FDA-2013-N-1317. *Federal Register*. 2015;80(116):34650–34670. Available at: https://www.gpo.gov/fdsys/pkg/FR-2015-06-17/pdf/2015-14883.pdf.

26. Fryar C, Carroll M, Ogden C. *Prevalence of Overweight, Obesity, and Extreme Obesity Among Adults: United States, 1960-1962 Through 2011-2012*. 2014. Available at: https://www.cdc.gov/nchs/data/hestat/obesity_adult_11_12/obesity_adult_11_12.pdf.

27. Centers for Disease Control and Prevention. Heart Disease Fact Sheet. 2016. Available at: http://www.cdc.gov/dhdsp/data_statistics/fact_sheets/fs_heart_disease.htm. Accessed November 11, 2016.

28. Schweikart L. *What Would The Founders Say?* New York: Penguin Group; 2011.

29. The Staff of the Select Committee on Nutrition and Human Needs United States Senate. *Dietary Goals for the United States*. Washington DC; 1977. Available at: http://zerodisease.com/archive/Dietary_Goals_For_The_United_States.pdf.

30. Burros M. In the Soda Pop Society-Can the American Diet Change for the Better? *Washington Post*. 1978:E1.

31. United States Congress. National Nutrition Monitoring and Related Research Act of 1990 (Public Law 101-445 - Oct. 22, 1990). 1990. Available at: https://www.gpo.gov/fdsys/pkg/STATUTE-104/pdf/STATUTE-104-Pg1034.pdf. Accessed September 22, 2016.

32. American Heart Association. The American Heart Association's Diet and Lifestyle Recommendations. *www.heart.org.* 2016. Accessed November 10, 2016.

33. Horowitz R. *Putting Meat on the American Table.* Baltimore: Johns Hopkins University Press; 2000:11–17.

34. Daniel C, Cross A, Koebnick C, Sinha R. Trends in meat consumption in the United States. *Public Health Nutrition.* 2011;14(4):575–583. Available at: https://www.ncbi.nlm.nih.gov/pmc/articles/PMC3045642/pdf/nihms-253312.pdf.

35. Wiest E. The Butter Industry In The United States: An Economic Study of Butter and Oleomargarine. In: The Faculty of Political Science of Columbia University, ed. *Studies in History, Economics and Public Law.* New York; 1916:202.

36. Ogden C, Carroll M, Fryar C, Flegal K. *Prevalence of Obesity Among Adults and Youth: United States, 2011-2014; No. 219.* Hyattsville; 2015. Available at: https://www.cdc.gov/nchs/data/databriefs/db219.pdf.

37. Centers for Disease Control and Prevention. Heart Disease Facts. *www.cdc.gov.* 2015. Available at: http://www.cdc.gov/heartdisease/facts.htm. Accessed September 23, 2016.

38. Grynbaum M. New York's Ban on Big Sodas Is Rejected by Final Court. *The New York Times.* 2014.

39. Sahadi J, Smith A. Philadelphia passes a soda tax. *www.money.cnn.com.* 2016. Available at: http://money.cnn.com/2016/06/16/pf/taxes/philadelphia-passes-a-soda-tax/.

40. Bjerga A, Bloomfield D. Tax on Sugary Foods Proposed by U.S. Panel to Fight Obesity. *Bloomberg.* 2015. Available at: http://www.bloomberg.com/news/articles/2015-02-19/tax-on-sugary-foods-proposed-by-u-s-panel-to-help-fight-obesity. Accessed September 23, 2016.

41. Lee B. 5 More Locations Pass Soda Taxes: What's Next for Big Soda? *www.forbes.com.* 2016.

42. Weiner J. Larry Summers: It's time to tax carbon and treats. *Washington Post.* 2012. Available at: https://www.washingtonpost.com/blogs/she-the-people/wp/2012/11/23/larry-summers-its-time-to-tax-carbon-and-treats/.

## Chapter 10:

1. Kleinfeldt R. How the Revolution Against Britain Divided Families and Friend. *The Making of A Nation.* Available at: http://www.manythings.org/voa/history/13.html. Accessed September 30, 2016.

2. Anon. Margaret Meda (1901-1978). *The Institute for Intercultural Studies.* Available at: http://www.interculturalstudies.org/Mead/index.html. Accessed June 7, 2015.

3. Lapin D. Personal Communication with Rabbi Lapin. 2016.

4. Kavanagh S. Don't put flame retardant chemicals in sports drinks! *change.org.* 2011. Available at: https://www.change.org/p/gatorade-don-t-put-flame-retardant-chemicals-in-sports-drinks. Accessed May 26, 2015.

5. Young S. Gatorade removes controversial ingredient after girl's online petition. *CNN.* 2013. Available at: http://eatocracy.cnn.com/2013/01/28/gatorade-removes-controversial-ingredient-after-girls-online-petition/comment-page-4/. Accessed May 26, 2015.

6. U.S. Food and Drug Administration. *Code of Federal Regulations Title 21: Sec. 180.30 Brominated vegetable oil.* 2015. Available at: http://www.accessdata.fda.gov/scripts/cdrh/cfdocs/cfcfr/cfrsearch.cfm?fr=180.30.

7. Zeratsky K. Should I be worried that my favorite soda contains brominated vegetable oil? *Mayo Clinic.* Available at: http://www.mayoclinic.org/healthy-lifestyle/nutrition-and-healthy-eating/expert-answers/bvo/faq-20058236. Accessed August 6, 2016.

8. Israel B. Brominated battle: Soda chemical has cloudy health history. *Environmental Health News.* 2011. Available at: http://www.environmentalhealthnews.org/ehs/news/2011/brominated-battle-in-sodas.

9. Mercola. Coca-Cola and PepsiCo Agree to Remove Flame Retardant Chemical from Their Products. *mercola.com.* 2015. Available at: http://articles.mercola.com/sites/articles/archive/2015/04/22/soda-flame-retardant-bvo.aspx.

10. Committee of Five. *Declaration of Independence.* Philadelphia; 1776. Available at: http://www.archives.gov/exhibits/charters/declaration_transcript.html.

## Chapter 11:

1. Grocery Manufacturer Association. GROCERY MANUFACTURERS ASSOCIATION POSITION ON GMOS. *The Facts About GMOs; A Project of The Grocery Manufacturers Association.* Available at: http://factsaboutgmos.org/disclosure-statement?_ga=1.19384190.792219552.1483234931. Accessed December 31, 2016.

2. Roseboro K. GMO labeling: Will grocery chains decide the issue? *www.newhope.com.* 2013. Available at: http://www.newhope.com/managing-your-retail-business/gmo-labeling-will-grocery-chains-decide-issue.

3. Weinberg C. What McDonald's Is Really Doing by Banning Antibiotics in Poultry. *www.eater.com.* 2015. Available at: http://www.eater.com/2015/3/11/8180183/mcdonalds-antibiotics-chicken-food.

4. Horovitz B. McDonald's not alone nixing antibiotics. *USA Today*. 2015. Available at: http://www.usatoday.com/story/money/2015/03/05/mcdonalds-antibiotics-fast-food-restaurants-chick-fil-a-tysons/24446801/.

5. Chipotle. G-M-Over It. *www.chipotle.com/gmo*. Available at: https://chipotle.com/gmo. Accessed November 10, 2016.

6. Velasco S. Panera Bread will remove all additives from its menu by 2016. Take that, Subway. *The Christian Science Monitor*. 2014.

7. U.S. Fish & Wildlife Service. Pollinators. *www.fws.gov*. 2016. Available at: https://www.fws.gov/pollinators/. Accessed August 22, 2016.

8. Center for Food Safety. Win for Democracy: Sonoma County Votes to Ban GMO Crops. *www.centerforfoodsafety.org*. 2016. Available at: http://www.centerforfoodsafety.org/press-releases/4569/win-for-democracy-sonoma-county-votes-to-ban-gmo-crops#. Accessed November 10, 2016.

9. Food & Water Watch. *rBGH How Artificial Hormones Damage the Dairy Industry and Endanger Public Health*. Washington DC; 2009. Available at: https://www.organicconsumers.org/sites/default/files/rbgh.pdf.

## Chapter 12:

1. Jeong MJ, Shim CK, Lee JO, et al. Plant gene responses to frequency-specific sound signals. *Molecular Breeding*. 2008;21(2):217–226.

## Permissions

*Chapter 11, Figure 1:* Non-GMO Project Verified butterfly seal. This material was reprinted with permission from the Non-GMO Project.

# INDEX

Made in United States
Orlando, FL
13 May 2022

17823909R00167